OLD

MAN

on a

BICYCLE

A Ride Across America and
How to Realize a More Enjoyable Old Age

OLD MAN

MAN

on a

BICYCLE

*A Ride Across America and
How to Realize a More Enjoyable Old Age*

DON PETTERSON

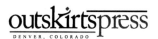
outskirtspress

DENVER, COLORADO

Old Man on a Bicycle
A Ride Across America and How to Realize a More Enjoyable Old Age

Outskirts Press, Inc.
http://www.outskirtspress.com

ISBN: 978-1-4787-2291-5

Outskirts Press and the "OP" logo are trademarks belonging to Outskirts Press, Inc.

Table of Contents

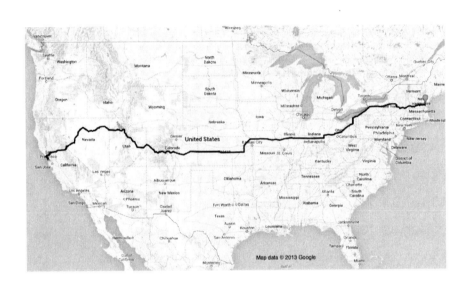

**Route—Brentwood, New Hampshire,
to San Francisco, California**

Prologue

Wispy streaks of cirrus clouds, floating six miles up in the cobalt sky above east-central Utah, provided no defense against the unrelenting sun. I had ridden over 100 miles the day before and figured that today's 64-mile ride between Green River and Price would be easy. But by noon the temperature had climbed almost to 100°, and the heat was sucking away my energy. The heat, an unexpectedly long climb, and a headwind for part of the morning had combined to make it a tough day. As I approached a turnoff into Price, where I would spend the night, I was thinking of the hot shower and subsequent cold beer I would soon be enjoying. At that moment, with no warning at all, I heard a loud whomp and simultaneously felt myself propelled forward by a tremendous force. Instinctively, I knew a car had hit me. Separated from the bike, I flew through the air, smacked into the ground, and rolled over several times before coming to rest. Lying there, stunned and unable to move, all I could do was wonder how badly I had been hurt.

PART I

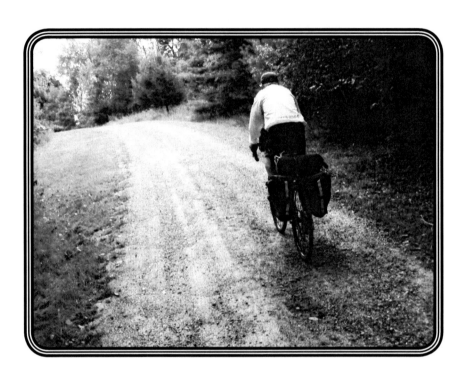

Heading West

CHAPTER 1

Outward Bound

Before the beginning of great brilliance, there must be chaos.

From the *I Ching*

The time had come for him to set out on his journey westward.

James Joyce

From my journal (at some point after ending each day's ride, I entered into a journal what I saw and did that day):

Day 1: Wednesday, May 8, 2002. Began the journey at 8:30, halted at 8:33. I noticed that the mini-computer[1] on my handlebars was on the fritz. Distracted by this while beginning to downshift to climb a steep incline on Pickpocket Road, a half mile from home, I managed to slip the chain and get it so badly jammed that I couldn't get it back on the ring. Made the first use of my cell phone by calling Julie to come pick me up in our mini-van. Went to Exeter Cycles, where one of the

---

1   Showing speed, distance traveled, time of day.

repair and maintenance crew adjusted the computer, showed me how to do it, dislodged the chain, and put it back on the ring. [This was not the first time I had slipped the chain, but it proved to be the last time, as I finally realized what I had been doing wrong.]

Under a mostly overcast sky and with the temperature at a pleasant 55°, I set out again. After three miles I turned west on NH Rte 27, where I encountered a light headwind that picked up after an hour or so. Nevertheless I made reasonably good time because the occasional hills on the way to Manchester weren't so bad. Only once did I have a problem—on Wellington Road going into the city, some 25 miles from home, a steep hill and wind gusts of up to 25 mph forced me to walk for a few minutes. Experienced my first city traffic while making my way through Manchester to the bridge across the Merrimac and found that riding in a city wasn't bad at all. Had a sandwich in Goffstown, about seven miles west of Manchester. The sky began to clear up and the temperature rose to the mid-60s.

For much of the time that afternoon I followed the course of a stream, passing through fields and woods. I stopped a couple of times to take pictures. The road to New Boston, Francestown, and Bennington was moderately hilly, and by 4 o'clock I was getting tired. So, when I found a motel three miles shy of the small New Hampshire town of Bennington I called it a day. Julie, Julianne, Jessica, and Samantha [respectively my wife, daughter, and granddaughters] drove from Exeter to meet me there later, and we went into town for dinner, after which we said our farewells and they went home. Writing this now, before I go to bed, I am a bit down, knowing that if all goes well I won't see Julie and the girls for a couple of months or so. But at the same time, I'm feeling good about having ridden a respectable distance this first day on the road.

Miles today = 58

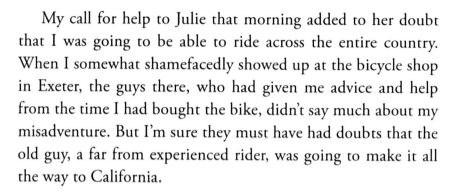

My call for help to Julie that morning added to her doubt that I was going to be able to ride across the entire country. When I somewhat shamefacedly showed up at the bicycle shop in Exeter, the guys there, who had given me advice and help from the time I had bought the bike, didn't say much about my misadventure. But I'm sure they must have had doubts that the old guy, a far from experienced rider, was going to make it all the way to California.

The bummer at the outset of my journey was a clear sign that I lacked experience and cycling smarts, which might have led a more prudent person to think twice about setting out to bicycle 3,000 or more miles. When I bought the bicycle and began training several months earlier, I hadn't been on one for many years. I got the bike in late September, and by the end of October temperatures had dropped to a point that I didn't want to continue riding. March 2002 was cold in New Hampshire, and it wasn't until early April that I found the weather warm enough to start riding again.

When I took off for San Francisco on May 8, my shortage of riding experience was evident: I was shaky on steep turns, had not practiced making emergency stops, and was clumsy when releasing my feet from the clamps on the bike's pedals as quickly as safety demanded. I could manage only the most basic repairs and knew nothing about making adjustments to, for example, the gear-shifting mechanism. Not only that, I had never made an overnight bike ride. And I hadn't yet built up enough muscular endurance.

Nevertheless, I didn't want to wait any longer, particularly since the earlier I began, the less summer heat I would encounter. Beyond that, I simply wanted to get going. Enough of training and preparing! The lure of the open road and the urge to begin were too strong to resist.

Seen from the vantage point of a spacecraft, the earth is not an immense place at all. Russian cosmonaut Valentina Tereshkova is widely quoted as having remarked, "Once you've been in space, you appreciate how small and fragile the Earth is." But, before setting out that cool, overcast May morning, I visualized an immense continent layered with countless hills and cross-hatched with north-south mountain ranges and vast plains extending far beyond western horizons. It was no wonder, given all this, that as I got on the bike and started out, my emotion was a mixture exhilaration and uncertainty.

Near the end of that first day, and throughout the second, I passed through southwestern New Hampshire's Monadnock region, an area of small towns, white-steepled churches, winding country roads lined with rock walls, covered bridges, forests, and hundreds of ponds and small lakes. Its hills and mountains had been created by glacial scouring of the last ice age, as the ice sheet that had reached as far south as Long Island made its retreat some 12,000 to 15,000 years ago. The region's hills are not too challenging for cyclists, and altogether the terrain made for a pleasant ride. Along with that, as the afternoon lengthened, the annoying headwind died down. It had turned out to be a beautiful day with a mainly clear sky and maximum temperature around 65°.

The lightly trafficked two-lane rural road through New Boston and Francestown on the way to Bennington took me past farmland and woods populated with oak, hickory, maple, beech, birch, and white pine. For almost an hour I rode alongside a clear stream dappled by sunlight reaching through the trees alongside it. Buoyed by the nice weather and the beauty around me, I easily put behind me both the embarrassing start and the struggle with the wind on the outskirts of Manchester. A good beginning after all.

CHAPTER 2

On Health, Aging and Adventure

Of all the self-fulfilling prophecies in our culture, the assumption that aging means decline and poor health is probably the deadliest.

Marilyn Ferguson, *The Aquarian Conspiracy*

Many people die at twenty-five and aren't buried until they are seventy-five.

Benjamin Franklin

Every human being is the author of his own health or disease.

Buddha

On a clear day, airline passengers flying across the country for the first time have a wondrous experience, as hypnotic views of the land several miles below slide by. But at the same time that they are afforded beautiful vistas of mountains and plains, lakes and deserts, and miniaturized cities and towns, they miss some dazzling scenery, such as the Niagara Falls, whose beauty is revealed only if seen up front and close.

Unlike those who are high in the sky, a cross-country bicyclist gets many marvelous close ups—for example, riding for miles alongside a rushing mountain stream or passing through deep forests. Yet, the scenic beauty is marred by warts-and-all aspects of roadside travel, such as trash thrown from cars, road kill, pieces of blown-out truck tires.

For me, another positive/negative feature of a bicycle trip became apparent as I proceeded slowly over the land: I met warm, friendly people, some of whom went out of their way to be helpful when help was needed; but I also had some encounters with hostile motorists who seemed to believe bicycle riders have no right to be on roads.

At times, I observed another contrast, one that I had seen a lot of before I rode across the country, as well as during the trip. On the one hand I saw people running or cycling or otherwise engaged in physical activity. But on the other hand I came across many who clearly showed that they had let poor eating habits and lack of exercise impair their health. I have an indelible image in my mind of stopping for lunch, parking my bike, and entering a restaurant in Delaware, Ohio, some 40 miles north of Columbus. Almost all the two dozen or so patrons were obese or noticeably overweight, about half were smoking, and most were plowing into large portions of food stacked high on their plates—a spontaneous, unrehearsed portrait of a perfect storm of bad health habits.

The rate that many Americans are eating and slouching their

way to serious medical problems by the time they reach middle age, some even earlier, is alarming. The Centers for Disease Control and Prevention reports that 36 percent of adults age 20 and over are obese and the combined percentage of obese and overweight adults is a shocking 69 percent, a marked increase over the past several decades. The increase has been accompanied by a rise in cases of diabetes, stroke, heart disease, and other health problems related to excessive weight. Some contend that the CDC's blanket is too wide, pointing out that it is a medical fact that being somewhat overweight is healthier than being underweight. Be that as it may, even if the percentage of at-risk people is not as high as reported by the CDC, there is no doubt that in this country, and some others as well—but as acute here as anywhere—there is an epidemic of corpulence that has medical consequences now and most likely will have even greater ones in the future.

And then there is tobacco usage. Although the percentage of adults who smoke has been halved over the past 50 years from 42 percent to 21 percent, about 45 million Americans (not including teenage smokers) are putting themselves at great risk to be afflicted by lung cancer, heart disease, or other smoking-related maladies.

Looking back over the past eight decades—my lifetime—I agree with any and all who have said that life is short. "It seems like only yesterday" may be a cliché, but to the old person who reminisces about days gone by it is a truism. As for the here and now, the older one gets, the faster time seems to glide by. In addition to that, not only is the dawning of a new day the first day of the rest of your life, it also means that another day of your allotted time on earth has ended. These observations lead to a conclusion that it makes eminent good sense to take care of yourself so that you can enjoy the days ahead as much as possible, and also that you should do all you can to influence the ones you love to take care of themselves.

At 83 I am in the ranks of the elderly, having graduated from the "young-old" cohort of those aged from 65 to 74 and moved into the "old-old" cluster, which ranges from 75 to 84. I am less than two years away from becoming one of the "oldest-old"—if, that is, I last that long. These may be artificial categories, but no matter how one looks at it, I am, whether I like it or not, an old man.

I'm highlighting my age at the outset of this book because *Old Man on a Bicycle* tells the tale of a septuagenarian's 3,600-mile bicycle trip, into which is woven a rejection of some of the generally accepted beliefs about aging and the resulting stereotyping of older people. (Sad but true, there is abundant evidence that some of the negativity stems from the attitudes of many over-65 men and women themselves.) And I offer authoritative, medically based suggestions for dealing with specific aspects of aging, such as a decrease in muscle mass.

According to the U.S. Census Bureau, in 2012 43 million Americans—about the population of Argentina or, closer to home, five million more than California's population—are 65 or older. That number is projected to increase dramatically in the next two decades, every day of which 10,000 baby boomers will reach age 65.

Four out of ten older Americans assess their health as very good or excellent. On the other hand, another four out of ten have a severe physical, sensory, or mental disability.

A high percentage of disabled older Americans can attribute their condition to past or current excesses, such as cigarette smoking, overeating, heavy drinking, or a sedentary life style. Of course many people are impaired through no fault of their own, drawing a genetic bad hand or being a victim of a debilitating or life-threatening disease or serious bodily injury. Stuff happens. Rather suddenly, or so it seemed to me, when I was 74 years old I was diagnosed with high blood pressure. Running a few times a week, beginning in my mid-40s, and doing some long-distance bicycle riding, starting in my early 70s, may have helped fend off the hypertension for a time, but did not stop its onset. High blood pressure evidently was lurking in my genetic makeup.

Many who are, or consider themselves to be, in mediocre or poor health, along with those whose health is good, can do a lot to improve their physical status and mental outlook. This requires, as a basis, a positive attitude toward aging. Those, whether young or old, who reflect on the aging process need to accept it and what it entails as an integral and natural part of the life cycle and certainly not as something to be feared. But, sad to say, fear and loathing of old age is an all too common attitude in this country; various studies have shown that Americans tend to view aging as a pathological process, a grim time of deterioration and decline.

As Betty Friedan pointed out in *Fountain of Aging*, "Clearly the image of age has become so terrifying to Americans that they do not want to see any reminder of their own aging."[2] She said a common view is that aging is a "problem" or a "plight"—a perception that, unfortunately, many older people buy into.

Low expectations, if not outright fears, lead many old people figuratively to curl up in a fetal position, to see no point in trying to remain physically and mentally vigorous. On the contrary, they make no effort to mitigate the unavoidable changes that come with aging, either not knowing or not believing that the vast majority of us can age more gracefully, with greater happiness, physical comfort, and sense of well-being.

Engaging in physical activity definitely can enhance physical functioning. Muscle strength, bone density, cardiovascular efficiency—all can be improved through exercise of one kind or another. A recent study found that "people are never too old to gain health benefits from exercise." Volunteers whose average age was 84 were divided into three groups, one of which exercised by walking, while another trained with weights, and a third did not exercise at all. After 16 weeks of regular exercise just twice a week, the first two groups "had lower systolic blood pressure, improved upper and lower body strength, improved hip and shoulder flexibility, and improvements in tests of agility, balance, and coordination when compared to the group that did not exercise."[3]

Less obvious, regular exercise can have a positive effect on depression, anxiety, and other psychological problems. Also, physical activity helps keep the aging brain fit, producing upswings in mental skills, memory retention, attention span, and

---

2   (New York: Random House, 1993), p. 41.

3   *New York Times*, February 28, 2006, D 5.

language skills.[4] Conversely, researchers have found that declines in physical activity cause deterioration of those attributes.

Other components of better health are well known: The *sine qua non* is, without a doubt, to stop smoking if you have not already done so, no matter what your age. In addition, a balanced diet that includes fewer calories and less saturated fat is essential for most people to better their prospects for good physical condition.

The message from health care experts is clear: If you are old or headed in that direction (if you're not, you've got a real problem), you should take a few simple steps to make your old age a better time for yourself and those who are close to you. If you are not in the best of health, those steps can actually lengthen your life, in the sense that your current habits could well be shortening it. If you are in reasonably good health, they most likely will not increase your life span, but, and this is he crux of what I'm saying, the quality of the time you have ahead of you will definitely improve. It's a question of personal choice, opting to exchange the probability of an unfulfilling, perhaps even miserable, old age for a future that allows you to retain or recapture at least some of the vigor that is so essential to living every day to its fullest.

All this is not to say that doing the right thing is a snap: Clearly, losing weight can be a tough undertaking, and many regard physical exercise as a pain in the butt. Therefore, essential components of a path to better health and a more palatable old age are commitment and self-discipline—a decision that

---

4 CB Taylor, JF Sallis, R Needle, "The Relation of Physical Activity an Exercise to Health," *Public Health Report*, 100 (Mar-Apr 1985): 195-202.

changed habits are absolutely necessary, and a determination to stick to a regimen that embodies those changes. Once having begun to exercise, many find that its physical and mental benefits are soon evident and so helpful that they become intent on making it a regular part of their life. A growing number of physicians recognize the medical value of exercise, particularly as a preventive health measure, and when appropriate advise their patients accordingly.[5]

What about considering possibilities that go beyond the basic ingredients of a healthy old age such as exercise and diet? What about pushing the edge of the envelope a bit? Here's where the idea of adventure comes in. I believe that life without an occasional adventure can, like a succession of cold, overcast, gray winter days, squeeze the soul.

Helen Keller once said: "Life is either a daring adventure or nothing."[6] While that may be overstating it for most people, the point is that venturing outside the ordinary can be a tonic. It's important to bear in mind that adventure can be defined in many ways and doesn't have to involve any risk. It needn't be more than some kind of change that provides an escape from the everyday demands of life and gives a boost to the spirit. Adventure, and

5   See, for example, Jordan Metzi, *The Exercise Cure* (New York: Rodale, 2013). One of the physicians who reviewed the book said it provides "compelling evidence for the important role [of exercise] in preventing and treating a number of diseases." Another writes: "Doctors have long focused on the treatment of disease. Now we have a manual that highlights a means of prevention. As Dr Metzl touts, exercise is one of the world's most effective medicines."

6   Helen Keller, *The Open Door* (New York: Doubleday, 1957) 17

whatever challenges or pleasures it offers is, in my opinion, another important component of an enjoyable old age.

For me, adventure took the form of a solo bicycle ride across the United States. Never having ridden more than several miles at a time, I didn't have a clue of what I was getting into. Ahead of me would be times when drenching cold rains, steep hills combined with headwinds, or physical pain would be more than I had bargained for. But there would also be sublime moments of awe as I slowly traversed a land whose beauty is at times breathtaking. And like many a lone traveler, certainly one on a bicycle, I would sometimes relish a feeling of absolute freedom.

CHAPTER 3

Before the Ride

Failure to prepare is preparing to fail.

Unknown

The secret of staying young is to live honestly, eat slowly, and lie about your age.

Lucille Ball

In the fall of 2001, I was two months short of turning 71 when I decided to try to cross America on a bicycle, even though I was not a cyclist. In fact, except for riding a few miles one day in Washington, DC, in the mid-1980s, I hadn't been on a bike since 1968, when I rode one to classes while I was at Stanford University, where, accompanied by Julie and our three children, I was on a fellowship. And a few years earlier, for several weeks I rode a bike to and from work at the American consulate in Zanzibar, the Indian Ocean island just off the east African coast. The last time before that would have been when I was an eighth grader delivering telegrams for Western Union in San Luis Obispo, California.

Like most boys in San Luis and in Pismo Beach, 12 miles to the south, where my family and I lived from 1933 to 1942, I had a bike. My first full-sized one was a Christmas present from my parents in 1940, after I had outgrown the second-hand, half-size model that I got when I was seven.

The new bike was a tan, white, and black Schwinn, complete with fenders. It had a battery-powered taillight and, attached to the handlebars, a small metal hemisphere-enclosed bell—the kind you rang by pulling on a lever that stuck out from its side. That first night I wheeled the bike out of the garage to the front of our house and turned on the taillight. The red glow that suffused the proximate darkness was, to me, a thing of rare beauty. Even today, more than 70 years later, in the same way that an odor triggered a memory in Proust's *Swan's Way,* sometimes a red light in a dark night rekindles that image in my mind.

But it wasn't a Proustian moment or sudden decision that led me to consider making an out of the ordinary journey across the continent. I was drawn to the idea for the most part simply because I figured it would be fun and stimulating. Perhaps because my time in the Foreign Service of the United States, which had included nine assignments to African countries, had been so eventful, at this quieter juncture in my life I was ready for some excitement. At first, I decided that I would like to fly across the country in an ultralight airplane. This thought came to me one day when I was mulling over what I might do after I finished writing my second book. A trans-America flight would be a cool (even 83-year-olds say "cool") way to return to California, where I was born and raised. An image of flying from New Hampshire to California in an ultralight got me excited, and I visualized taking off and heading west, with the whole country—mountains, plains, farmland, rivers—unfolding beneath me.

It wasn't that I hadn't been to California since leaving in 1960 to join the Foreign Service. Over the years I had returned there many times with Julie and our children, visiting family and friends on home leave between assignments abroad. We also spent an academic year at Stanford, where I had received a fellowship, and later a year at UCLA, where the State Department assigned me as a diplomat in residence. But I found I was still drawn to return yet again.

In 1996 Ninja, a tomcat, after being moved by his owners from the state of Washington to a new home in Utah, 850 miles away, disappeared, only to turn up at his old home a year later. Salmon swim upriver to spawn in the very stream where they were born. This they do after having lived hundreds or even thousands of miles away in the ocean, guided, some scientists say, by smell alone; others say the fish are tuned in to, and guided by, the Earth's magnetic force field. The migrations of birds over thousands of miles back to where they were hatched is no less amazing for being well known and exhaustively studied. Diverse facts and theories have been advanced to attempt to explain how these and other creatures find their way back, but in essence there is something in their brain that enables them to "remember" how to return to where they originated. It seems that humans do not have a cerebral component to match the homing instinct of animals. But something in us draws us back, if not to where we were born, certainly to where we were raised.

It is not uncommon when having returned to a place where

you lived years before to find that it is quite different from what you remembered. Sometimes the changes are so profound that going back is a shock or at least a deep disappointment. And yet not everything changes, and returning home can trigger strong feelings of being linked with a past that may be gone but is nevertheless very real in our memories. Calvin Weisberger, a Los Angeles cardiologist, put it well when he wrote:

We all carry a component of where we came from in our personalities. We all have behavior that is shaped by our early life experiences. Wherever we come from, whatever our home is like, we carry it with us. As we carry fond memories of beloved people, we can carry fond memories of home, whatever it has become. Perhaps in the end, home is not so much a place as an idea.[7]

In addition to the appeal of an adventure and responding again to the pull of California, I had a notion, goofy though it may have been, that an out-of-the-ordinary passage to California would in a sense be like the journeys of my ancestors who had migrated from the eastern United States to California in the 19th century. One of my great-grandfathers on my mother's side, a ship's officer from Maine, had, on his last voyage, sailed from Boston to San Francisco via Cape Horn. The other maternal great-grandfather, also from Maine, took a ship to Panama, crossed the Isthmus, and sailed on up to California. And one of my maternal great-grandmothers was born in Soda Springs, Utah Territory, in 1854. Her parents, who had left Pennsylvania, were traveling west in a covered-wagon train headed for Washington.

---

7   "You Can't Go Home," *The Permanente Journal* 6, No. 4 (Fall 2002), 69.

One cool, clear late-August morning of 2001, I drove from my town of Brentwood in southeastern New Hampshire to a flying field west of Concord near the Vermont border to take a ride in a fixed-wing ultralight.

A half-century earlier, when I was an enlisted man in the navy, after more than two years of sea duty I was transferred to the US naval air station at Corpus Christi, Texas, where, as an aerographer (the navy's term for meteorologist) I was required to fly occasionally as a weather observer. Although I was glad to get flight pay and enjoyed the flights once in the air, before and during takeoffs I had sweaty palms and a nervous stomach. A buddy of mine at the air station, a licensed pilot, encouraged me to watch some training films for fledgling navy pilots and think about learning to fly. His encouragement and the films did the trick, and I resolved to confront my fear of flying by taking flying lessons.

When I was off duty I went to Cudahy Field, a privately owned airport near Corpus Christi, and began going up with an instructor. In March 1952 I soloed and in June I got my license. I flew in the area near Corpus Christi and around southern Texas until I was discharged in July. I kept flying now and then when I was a student at the University of California, Santa Barbara, making flights in a flying club's Aeronca Champion, a single engine airplane in the same league as a Piper Cub. Naturally, I showed off, buzzing Santa Barbara's East Beach, where college kids hung out. Once, to impress Helen, a gorgeous co-ed whom I was dating, I took her on a short hop over Santa Barbara. This turned out to be a big mistake, for Helen got airsick.

My flying career, such as it was, came to a close while I was in gradate school because my undergraduate scholarship had ended, I had run out of GI Bill benefits, and my income from part-time jobs wasn't enough to allow me the luxury of renting an airplane. Until that August morning in the sky over New Hampshire, some 45 years later, I had assumed that my flying skills would be easy to revive and that it would be a simple matter to fly an ultralight. But I was wrong. During the flight, when the pilot let me take the controls I found that although the basic mechanics of controlling the aircraft, such as turning, banking, and maintaining altitude, were the same as those I had used in flying years before, my skills were worse than rusty, the handling characteristics of the ultralight were subtly different, and landing it was not the same as landing the airplanes I had flown.

Low airspeed is crucial to the usual procedure for landing a single-engine light airplane not having a tricycle landing gear (e.g., a Piper Cub). With the power cut, you come in slow, level off a few feet above the runway, raise the nose to reduce speed even more and, if you do it right, stall out just as the two wheels of the landing gear and the tail wheel touch the ground simultaneously. This could not be done in the kind of aircraft in which I was flying that morning because at low speed the ultra-light's controls became mushy and didn't respond well to movement of the stick or rudder pedals. As a result, it was necessary to come in fast, and that, as I will explain, was more than interesting.

Unlike the airplanes I had flown, the basic ultralight has no enclosed cabin. The wing of the plane I flew in that morning was above and just behind pilot and passenger, and the motor and propeller were aft of the wing. The landing gear consisted of a small nose wheel and two other small wheels protruding on slender tube-like struts from the airframe. The distance between the bucket seat in which I sat and the ground when the aircraft was at rest or taxiing was only about a foot. As a consequence, when the plane swooped in to land at 50 miles an hour or so with me perched on its forward end, I could be forgiven for feeling like a witch on the front end of a large broomstick.

Flying in the ultralight was exciting. But as much as I liked it, I began to have second thoughts about using one of them for a cross-country journey. Not only were my flying skills so badly corroded that I would have to take a good number of lessons to become a proficient pilot, but also there was the not inconsiderable cost of buying an ultralight to consider. I decided to think it over.

After a day or two, I dropped the idea of flying to California. And in the moment that I did, for some reason—I'm not sure why—it occurred to me that instead of flying I could ride a bicycle. With no conception whatsoever of what this would entail, I thought it would be worth pursuing. Had I known just how grueling some of the days on the road would turn out to be, I might have opted to take a Greyhound bus. But insulated from reality by my ignorance, before long I decided I would give it a shot.

I said nothing about this to Julie. Then one day in early September when she and I were having lunch with a close friend at a restaurant overlooking Flathead Lake in Montana, the conversation took a turn that led me to tell our friend that I intended to ride a bike across the US. Julie was both surprised and incredulous.

"You're kidding," she said.

"No I'm not; I'm serious."

"You're crazy! You can't do that; it's impossible."

"Why not?"

"You don't even have a bicycle."

Our friend just laughed. When Julie realized I was serious, knowing how stubborn I could be and that continuing to tell me it was not possible would just make me dig in my heels even deeper, she let the matter drop. There are times when told something I want to do is not a smart move, I tend to react like, "What do you mean I can't do it; by gosh, I'll show you," or some such silly macho/adolescent declaration.

Not wanting any flak from family or friends, I pretty much kept my plan close to my vest. One person had faith in me, my best friend, Bruce McCurdy. At UC Santa Barbara we had shared an apartment for a year, worked one summer as laborers at a building construction site, and were primed to drop whatever we were doing and embark on an "adventure," however we interpreted it. In the Aeronca, with Bruce serving as navigator, we flew north from Santa Barbara to places like San Luis Obispo and Bakersfield. One of our extra-curricular projects was to build a raft, which promptly sank when we launched it in the ocean. Whenever we could we played golf—pewee golf, that is; we could neither afford the cost nor devote the time needed to play regular golf.

When Julie and I were in Santa Barbara on the same trip that had taken us to Montana, we spent time with Bruce, who by then was a retired art professor at UCSB, and his wife, Beverly. After I told them what I was thinking of doing, Bruce thought it was a great idea. He was so enthusiastic about what he saw as another adventure we could do together that he volunteered to accompany me in his mini-van and provide whatever support I might need. He really meant it, even though fully aware that it would mean many days sitting in his car waiting for me to complete the day's ride. But it was not to be, for unfortunately soon afterward Bruce became ill and physically unable to make the trip.

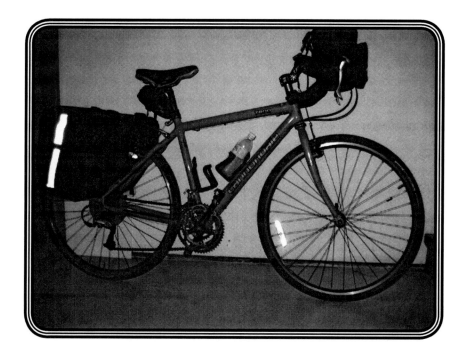

My Cannondale

In mid-September of that year, 2001, a month after I had dropped the idea of flying an ultralight, I bought a touring bike—a

Cannondale T-800—in Exeter, a town that abuts Brentwood, and equipped it with a rack on the back, two rear panniers (saddle-bags), and a handlebar bag. Touring bicycles are heavier than the more popular road bicycles, their heavier frame enabling them to carry loads too heavy for road bikes. A longer wheelbase, sturdier wheels, and wider tires are also features of the bike's greater load-bearing capacity. And compared to road bikes' single mount for water, touring bikes have as many as three.

For an old geezer, I was in pretty good shape, mainly because I had been a runner since my early forties. But I knew I would have to strengthen different muscles to ride a bicycle and develop the necessary endurance to keep going for hours at a time on successive days. My first task, though, was to learn basic skills, like shifting, using hand brakes, getting accustomed to clip-in pedals, riding in town traffic, removing wheels, and changing tire tubes. While still getting the hang of these, I rode through Exeter one day. Spying some friends walking on the other side of the street, I waved and came to a sudden halt. As I did so, I was unable to unclip my feet from the pedals quickly enough, and the bike and I flopped to the pavement. Embarrassed, after assuring them I was all right, I continued my ride. My injuries were a scraped forearm and a bruised ego.

I began building up mileage, trying to take care not to overdo it at first. As I added to the distance of my rides, I had to cope with saddle soreness. I knew this was likely to happen until I got used to riding, but the discomfort was more than I expected, in part, I suppose, because I'm not at all well padded, posteriorily speaking. I ended up trying several different saddles, and in fact it wasn't until I reached Colorado that I finally settled on the saddle that I would use from then on.

In making preparations, I did little in the way of advance planning beyond laying out a tentative course from New Hampshire to San Francisco, gathering road maps, seeking advice from a couple of state departments of transportation, reading a few accounts on the Internet by cyclists who had made long-distance rides, and checking with some of them and with a number of cycling clubs about road conditions in their area. Because I hadn't laid out an exact route, I didn't search the Internet to locate bicycle shops along the way or to determine which towns would be sure to have places to stay. As it happened, I lucked out and almost always came across bike shops when I needed them and managed to find overnight accommodations as I rode along. Before setting out on later trips, however, I did check the Internet to locate bicycle shops and motels along my route. This added a welcome degree of certainty to those trips.

Initially I planned to camp part of the time and carried a tent, sleeping bag, and other items for camping. There's no question that camping saves money, and the rider on a tight budget would probably opt for it. There are, though, two major downsides to camping that the rider who can afford the expenses of motels and restaurants should bear in mind. First, campers must carry extra weight—camping gear, food, and a cooking utensil or two. Younger, stronger riders may not care about that weight, but the older crowd, which obviously includes me, might be inclined to travel as lightly as possible. Second, the campground experience may not appeal to everyone. I, for one, wanted peace and quiet at night and the assurance of a good night's sleep. Campgrounds can be noisy, and in the late spring and the summer in northerly parts of the country they do not get dark until after 9 pm and quiet until later than that. These two disadvantages would figure in my thinking as I rode west through New Hampshire, southern Vermont, and upstate New York. When I'd been on the road for about a week, I decided to send my camping gear home.

After I ditched the tent and other camping items, my load, which included what I wore, consisted of:

2 spandex bike shorts

1 pair tights

1 pair khaki trousers

1 pair semi-waterproof running pants

1 cotton and 2 wick-dry-material T-shirts

1 long-sleeve T, wick-dry material

1 short-sleeve sport shirt (for evening wear)

1 sweatshirt

1 lightweight lime-green windbreaker

1 pair walking shorts

3 handkerchiefs

3 pair white sox

1 pair cycling shoes

1 pair sneakers

Cycling gloves, helmet, sun glasses

Baseball cap

Warm gloves for cold weather

A sleeping bag (for emergency use)

2 spare tubes, 1 tire-patching kit

Hand pump, tire lever, chain oil, cleaning rag,
    2 Allen wrenches, 4 bungee cords

Small pair of pliers

Bicycle combination cable lock

Pocketknife

Camera

Cell phone and charger cable

3" x 5" radio and headphone

Steno pad and pen for trip journal

Road maps

Paperback book

Chamois butter anti-chafing lubricant

Sunscreen, toothpaste and brush, razor, dental floss, sham-
    poo, band-aids, anti-inflammatory pills, antibiotic
    ointment

2 water bottles

Spare cash, credit card, ATM card, phone card, ID

I also carried a battery-operated small taillight and a flashlight, which, for the infrequent times I needed forward illumination, I attached to the handlebar bag with duct tape. Opting for a minimum-weight load, I did not bring spare spokes or a spare tire. And since water or other liquids, such as Gatorade, were the heaviest items in my load, each day I carried as few filled replenishment bottles as I could safely get by with, the number depending on how hot the day was going to be and how far I would be riding between places where I could buy more if I needed them.

A practical thought that occurred to me was to pack most of my load into large Ziploc bags to keep things dry when it rained. Using this procedure also made it easier for packing and unpacking at the beginning and end of each day's ride.

Every morning, I would try to start out with bananas and/or power bars in my handlebar bag, either to help keep me going until I could get breakfast when there was none at the motel or for energy between meals on the road.

My minimalist approach to what I would carry on the bike arose from the knowledge that I would be climbing the Appalachians, Rockies, and Sierras, not to mention some formidable hills in between. Riders not as concerned about weight as I was will, no doubt, find my list of what to carry deficient in one respect or another. But it worked fine for me.

By early November, temperatures had dropped to the point that I didn't want to continue riding. But before the winter settled in, I had increased the distance of my longest training ride to 55 miles. Over the winter I worked out at a local gym on a stationary bike either at a spin class or by myself. And I ran a few times a week, three to six miles each run, unless the roads were too icy. March 2002 was cold in New Hampshire, and it wasn't until early April that I found the weather warm enough to start riding. By the end of the month I had increased my longest ride to 70 miles and had made a 50- and a 60-mile ride back to back. I was ready to go, but before I could start my cross-country ride I joined Julie in Mexico for a few days to attend the celebration of her mother's 85th birthday. I get along well with my Mexican relatives, and Julie says they hold me in high regard. Nevertheless, their reaction to my plan was similar to hers:

"¡Estás loco, Don!" *(You're crazy, Don!)*

¿En qué piensas?" *(What in the world are you thinking?)*

"Oye, tu eres muy viejo para tratar de hacer un viaje tan lejos en bicicleta."

(Hey, you're too old to try to make such a long trip on a bicycle.)

And other expressions of disbelief. But of course they wished me Godspeed and urged me to be as careful as I could.

If my four children, Susan (39), Julianne (38), John (36), and Brian (22), doubted that I was capable of riding three thousand or more miles, they never expressed it. Instead, all four said, in essence, "Go for it, Dad!"

Julie and I returned to New Hampshire on May 5. I got in a couple of rides, made final preparations, and on the 8th began my westward journey.

CHAPTER 4

New Hampshire and Vermont

Anything I can say about New Hampshire
Will serve almost as well about Vermont,
Excepting that they differ in their mountains.
The Vermont mountains stretch extended straight;
New Hampshire mountains curl up in a coil.

Robert Frost

After that satisfactory first day on the road and a good night's sleep, I was eager to resume the ride. The weather didn't look too promising, but the rain that was falling when I started eased into a drizzle then ended completely after an hour or so.

From my journal:

Day 2: Thursday, May 9. Departed at 7:45 in moderate rainfall, headed for Brattleboro, Vermont. Took a couple of wrong turns but got straightened out, I thought, by getting directions from a motorist. Unfortunately his advice just led me further astray. When I saw a light on at a house, I stopped and knocked on the door. It was opened

33

by a sleepy-looking man of about 50, who, not at all irritated by being awakened, wanted to know where I has headed. When I told him California, he said, "Wow, hope you make it," and told me how to get to the nearest town, Hancock, which I reached in less than half an hour. It was about 9, and I was getting hungry but didn't see an open café or restaurant. Still unsure which way to go, I left town and ended up on back roads that took me in a westerly direction over hill country and by a lovely small lake into Harrisville about an hour later. Still navigating by guess and by gosh, I went south four miles to Dublin, where to my joy, for I was starving, I finally found a café at 11. Until then I'd subsisted on two bananas and some Gatorade. Had great pancakes, bacon, and orange juice.

From Dublin west to Keene was mostly downhill, which made up for the steep hills I had encountered earlier. By NH standards Keene, with some 23,000 residents, is one of the state's larger towns. In comparison Hancock, Harrisville, and Dublin have populations in the neighborhood of 1,500. I got lost, yet again, on the outskirts of Keene, and found myself heading south. Realized this was a bad move, went back, and found the correct route, NH 9, to Brattleboro, Vermont. More hills, but the terrain leveled off near Brattleboro, where I am overnighting at a hotel.

From here to Albany the route is uncomplicated (only one road— Vermont 9, which morphs into NY 7) so there won't be a repeat of today's meanderings. I'm comfortably tired tonight, if I can put it that way, but in any case, the 57 miles from Bennington to Brattleboro have added to my optimism that I can do this thing.

57 miles = 115 total mileage

Riding a bike for hours at a time burns lots of calories, just how many depends on circumstances, in particular the shape of the land, wind direction and force, and amount of weight carried. According to one expert, 5,000 to 10,000 calories is a ballpark figure for the amount that would be consumed on a single full day's bike ride. Even at the low end of the estimate, that means a lot of food has to be ingested. One benefit for those who have to watch their weight is that when riding a long distance, by and large there is no need to be concerned about eating too many carbohydrates or too much fat (as long as it isn't trans fat).

It is axiomatic, then, that cross-country riders need a hearty breakfast at the outset of the day or as soon as possible after getting underway. This sometimes was a problem for me. There would be days, like the second one of my trip, when, there being no place to eat where I had spent the night, I would ride for a good part of the morning before finding a restaurant. Because of this, good sense dictated that I had something like donuts or bananas or energy bars on hand to eat before I left my room or while looking for someplace to get a regular breakfast.

The distances traveled each of those first two days were nothing great, but not too bad considering the hills, the unfavorable winds, and that I was not yet as strong as I should have been. In Brattleboro, my only stop in Vermont, after getting settled in a hotel room in town, I nursed two beers at a tavern while watching the Red Sox play Oakland, had dinner, was in bed with a book by 9:30, and asleep about an hour later. I confess that I was so intent on keeping my bike load to a minimum that as I progressed through the paperback book I was reading, I tore out the pages I had finished.

My end-of-ride pattern was already set: Get a room; wheel the bike inside; unpack what I needed from the panniers; wash bike shorts, t-shirt, socks, and handkerchief; shower; have a beer; eat dinner; lay out what gear I would need for the next day's ride; and repack the panniers, check out the Weather Channel's forecast, and maybe watch something else on TV, read, and hit the sack. Every few days I would clean parts of the bike and wipe off and re-oil the chain. I later learned that I probably should have cleaned and re-oiled the chain more often.

On this trip, only once, at the hotel in Brattleboro, was I unable to take my bike into my room. Unsure about the protocol on this, I agreed to park the bike in an enclosure in the lobby. Had I known that this was an unusual requirement, and that my departure could be delayed, I would not have stayed there but instead would have found some other place to spend the night.

From the journal:

Day 3: Friday, May 10. Have had a great ending to a sometimes-hellacious day. Awoke at 5:30 and could have started by 6:30, but since the desk clerk, who had the key to the bicycle enclosure in the lobby, didn't arrive until 8, I didn't get underway until about 8:30. Began climbing even before leaving town. Had breakfast at a café at mile five (very soggy pancakes). I had been carrying a second saddle, switching the two now and then to see which was more comfortable. Choosing one as I exited the café, I left the other on a ledge near the entrance, not wanting to carry the extra weight, and then began a long struggle with a 15-20 mph headwind with gusts, according to the Weather Channel, of as much as 40 mph. About two miles from the café, a car passed me and pulled to a stop. The man and woman in the car flagged me down. They said they had seen me in the café, spotted the saddle, figured it was mine and that I'd forgotten it, and set out to chase me down. I groaned inwardly, but thanked them profusely. After they drove off, I decided maybe it was providential that the saddle had been returned to me, and decided to keep it. I strapped it on the rack holding the panniers and continued the climb.

The 19-mile ascent against the wind and up some steep inclines was so tough that I had to dismount and walk briefly four times. Twice, when I was riding at three or four mph, a sudden strong gust of wind blew me over, whammo, on my left side, which was better for the bike, for no damage was done to the chain rings or derailleurs [which are on the right side], but a bit scary because I fell a wee bit into the roadway. At long last I reached the summit and experienced the exhilaration of coasting for several miles on the descent. Because the loaded panniers might have destabilized the bike coasting at high speed, and also because of my inexperience in going downhill at such a fast clip, I used the brakes to keep the velocity at no more than 36 mph.

At around 4 pm I reached Hoosick, New York, a few miles from the Vermont-New York border, only to find no motel, no campground, no food store. An elderly woman standing by the walkway to her house told me she thought there might be a motel two or three miles farther on. Considering that she seemed to be a native, it was odd that she didn't know for sure if there was a motel up the road. But anyway, there it was, near the top of a fairly steep grade and next-door to a tavern, to which, after my daily ritual of showering, *washing clothes, etc., I repaired to enjoy a draft beer and excellent fish and chips. Had good conversation with the bartender and two women patrons, who wanted to know about my journey and ended up getting the story of my life. After I'd told them where I was headed, they expressed amazement and seemed even more blown away when I mentioned how old I am. I have to say I get a kick out of playing the old-man card. The cost of the motel room was $51, tax included, [about the average that I spent on overnight accommodations on the trip]. Considering the mornings strenuous climbing, I'm satisfied with today's total of 54 miles.*

54 miles = 160 total

Today's ride was a rigorous test of my staying power. It involved two climbs, the first beginning not far out of Brattleboro and rising for about 15 miles to Hogback Mountain. This segment was the more difficult of the two, even though, except for a few tough short spells, it wasn't all that steep. However, for most of its 15 miles it steadily ascended before more or less leveling off then descending a short way into the small town of Wilmington. The second climb, starting a few miles from Wilmington, was steeper but a lot shorter. By itself, the 19-mile ascent would have been tough, but coupled with the unrelenting headwind, it almost undid me, and I very much welcomed the restful descent into Bennington.

Making it a point to let my new friends in the tavern know my age was a far cry from my initial sentiments about getting old. Over the years I'd gotten used to being told that I looked young for my age, and I never tired of hearing it. Pure vanity, I know, but there are worse sins. It's not that I tried to deny to myself the reality of my age. For example, after reaching 60, I had not suddenly gone in for dying my hair, piercing parts of my body, wearing a big gold chain around my neck, getting a tattoo, or buying the latest mod fashions. Nothing like that. But I was uncomfortable about joining the ranks of the elderly, which I suppose is a comment on how much I was influenced by how old people are generally regarded in our society.

One day, when Julie and I and our youngest child, Brian, then three and a half years old, were on home leave in 1983 after leaving Somalia, where I had been the American ambassador for four years and where Brian had been born, we went to a restaurant in Santa Cruz, California. While we were waiting to be seated, a sixtyish woman looked at Brian and said to me, "You have an adorable grandchild." I was 52 at the time, and no doubt looked more like a grandfather than a father of a small child. Instead of being amused, as I should have been, I was chagrined by the lady's well-meaning observation.

As I got well into my sixties, I was at peace with neither the concept nor the reality of being an old person, even though I was well aware that time will have its way with the body. An object lesson in that regard occurred when I was 41, in Freetown, Sierra Leone. Playing on the embassy's basketball team, I was in fairly good shape, but playing full-court basketball was killing me. The back and forth on offense and defense, which I handled well enough when I played on my junior college team less than 20 years earlier, was so physically demanding that it was downright painful. However, there was no way that I, in charge of the embassy at the time, could throw in the towel. So I persevered until one night when we were playing a Sierra Leone army team, I caught a pass poorly, jamming a finger and badly spraining it. I accepted commiserations from players on both sides, as it was clear I was finished for the season. I appeared saddened by this, but inwardly I was exultant—I wouldn't have to play any more.

Perhaps like a lot of us, despite getting up in years, in my sixties and into my seventies I didn't feel aged nor did I visualize myself as such. However, mirrors and physical realities, like stiffening joints, intruded and after a while I came to accept what I was. Preparing for and making the ride across the country helped change my perspective, and I began almost to revel in my senescence. Well, not quite. But during the trip I was amused when people seemed startled to learn how old I was when the subject of my age came up during their questions about where I was coming from and where I was headed.

Not only have I accepted being old, but I've come to enjoy some aspects of old age, such as having grandchildren, being relieved of the stresses of a competitive career, having time do things I couldn't do during my working life, and more intensely valuing my friendships and personal relationships.

There is a flip side to acceptance of old age: There are those who, in their sixties or older or even only in their fifties, act in ways that fit a stereotype of old people. Some put undue limits on physical activities that they mistakenly consider beyond their capacity or even harmful. While perhaps it is natural to like being with persons more or less your own age, some carry this to an extreme, voluntarily avoiding interaction with younger people.

My bicycling inexperience had been apparent again on this day's ride, when my body abruptly met the pavement, not once, but twice. There are times—an unexpected sudden encounter with sand on a sharp curve in a road, for instance—when even skilled cyclists can lose control. As for me, though, if I had ridden a lot more to prepare for the trip, I would have had a better feel for how to avoid a fall. And I would likely have been better able to execute a quick release from the pedal clamps. Looking at the flops from a positive angle, I didn't break any bones. And therein lies a lesson.

The process of bone formation and bone loss goes on throughout life. Bone loss, or resorption, occurs through the breakdown and assimilation of bone tissue by the action of cells called osteoclasts. Obviously, as a child grows, formation surpasses loss. Between the time when growth stops, at around age 18, until about age 35 on average, there is a balance between formation and loss, and bone strength is stable. From then on, however, bone loss gradually surpasses formation, resulting in a slow reduction of bone mass (density). This is an unavoidable aspect of aging. But it needn't be a sentence to fragility or debilitating osteoporosis.

The best defense against being cursed with excessively weakened bones in later years is to build strong bones before age 30. All the young people who read this book—all six of them, if you count my grandchildren—should take note of this. Gaining the maximum bone mass through exercise and proper nutrition during childhood, adolescence, and young adulthood is a major factor in the prevention of osteoporosis, a disease in which the bones become extremely porous, are subject to fracturing spontaneously or by minimal trauma, and heal slowly.

An estimated ten million Americans suffer from osteoporosis and another 34 million have low bone mass, the precursor osteoporosis. That's an astonishing number, given that most of this could have been prevented, although perhaps not at all astonishing when you consider the extent of another preventable epidemic in this country, obesity. In any event, it's a no-brainer to recognize that a healthy lifestyle can be critically important to keeping bone loss to a minimum.

To be specific, whether or not you have built up maximum bone mass during your formative years, there are a few simple steps that favor bone strength. Get out and about on sunny days because vitamin D, which is needed to promote the absorption of calcium, is synthesized in the body by exposure to sunlight (but of course take care to avoid overexposure, which can do serious damage to the skin). In addition, eat plenty of calcium rich food, such as yogurt, milk, cheese, salmon, spinach, broccoli, peas, and calcium-fortified breakfast cereals. Forsake the life of a couch potato and adopt a program of regular exercise because, as important as a proper diet is, without exercise it won't do the trick of sustaining bone strength as we grow older. Just like real estate agents' assertion that "location, location, location" is key to a property's value, "exercise, exercise, exercise" is critical to good health. Had I not engaged in one form or another of exercise—tennis, squash, walking, running—over the years, I might not have been fit enough to ride across the country, and I could easily have broken a hip or other bone when I fell to the pavement.

Vermont Rte 9W from Brattleboro to Bennington (Vermont—there's another Bennington in New Hampshire) crosses the southernmost extent of the Green Mountains, themselves near the northern end of the Appalachians, which are among the oldest mountains in the world. At its highest point, the highway never exceeded 3,000 feet, so altitude was not a challenge. But, starting at Brattleboro, with its 240-foot elevation, the winding road climbs to well over 2,000 feet and includes some steep gradients that, combined with this day's headwinds, gave me considerable grief. Balancing this, the several miles of downhill coasting and the impressive view south from Hogback Lookout of forested rows of hills extending into Massachusetts were enjoyable. And having ridden up and over the mountain range gave me a sense of accomplishment.

For the third day in a row at this outset of the journey, stymied by strong, gusting winds as I was climbing particularly steep inclines, I had to get off the bike and walk with it for a spell. Over-achiever that I am, I was chagrined to have to do this. Now, looking back, I realize that my legs were not yet as strong as they ultimately would become, but that even if they had been, the day's combination of wind and hills would still have made it very difficult to keep riding safely during the climbs. In the days ahead, I would be forced to dismount only once more, 43 days later west of Gunnison, Colorado.

CHAPTER 5

New York and Pennsylvania

To me, old age is always 15 years older than I am.

Bernard M. Baruch

The wind doth blow today, my love

Unknown

From the journal:

Day 4: Saturday, May 11. Another day apparently designed to test my will and to make me wonder why the hell I am doing this. Rte 9 in Vermont had become New York Rte 7, and I followed it to Troy. In the 20-odd miles to Troy there were only a few moderate climbs and they alternated with some restful downhills. But, damnation, the westerly headwind was still blowing—20 mph with gusts up to who knows how much. In Troy I augmented my PowerBar and banana breakfast with eggs, bacon, and toast at a diner. Thanks to the great directions I had received in an email from the NY Department of Transportation, I had no problem negotiating the crossing of the Hudson, the south turn into

*and through downtown Albany, and then the turn to the west onto US
20. Once headed west, I was slowed again by the bloody wind. Had a
hot dog at a Lion's Club trailer just outside a town called Duanesburg.
The man in the trailer told me that there would be no place to stay on
US 20 for at least another 15 miles. I'd gone 50 miles at this point
and was tired of fighting the wind, which at times slowed me down
to five mph on level stretches. Advised that there was a Holiday Inn
eight or nine miles down the road on NY Rte 7, which at Duanesburg
intersected with US 20 again, branching off in a west-southwest direction, I elected to look for it. <u>Eleven</u> hard miles later, I arrived at the
Holiday Inn, only to find that there were no vacancies. Taking pity on
me, a clerk called around and finally found an opening at a motel at
Cobleskill, only a few miles away.*

61 miles = 230 total

I remember that when I was a kid it seemed that much of the
time the wind was against me when I rode my bike into town
and against me when I rode back home. As for the cross-country
trip, time and again in my journal I complain about headwinds.
I came to see the wind more often than not as antagonistic,
a malicious creature waiting to pounce and take a chunk out
of me. Surfing the Internet shows that among cyclists I'm far
from alone in my odium for adverse winds; I found that wind
is the number one bête noir of serious bicycle riders. Even a
light breeze blowing against a cyclist can significantly reduce
the speed of forward motion. A stronger wind, say one that cuts

the rider's average speed in half or more, is discouraging, to say the least. And having to pedal downhill to maintain forward progress is no fun.

The prevailing upper wind pattern in the continental United States is from west to east, and as any frequent cross-country flier knows, it takes more time to fly from the East Coast to the West Coast than vice-versa. However, on the surface of the earth, mountains and other topographical features, the relative positions of low- and high-pressure air masses, and differences in heating and atmospheric pressure cause variations in the west-east pattern. That notwithstanding, the conventional wisdom is that a cross-country cyclist is well advised to ride from west to east. Most commercial bicycle tours do it that way, as did the authors of almost all the articles or books I read about riding from one end of the country to the other.

However, I wanted to go from east to west, to start out where I live, just 13 miles west of the Atlantic Ocean, ride in the same general direction that some of my ancestors had traveled a century and a half or so ago, and end in San Francisco. Had I known how much strong westerly winds would pummel me during a good portion of the journey, I might have had second thoughts about which direction I should take. The mix of the headwinds and hills I encountered in the first few days of the ride tested my resolve to keep going and were harbingers of some tough days ahead.

Between the 8th of May and the 31st, I struggled with head-winds 11 days and had trouble with crosswinds three, a total of 60 percent of the time. That pretty much confirmed the conventional wisdom. However, for the rest of the journey, headwinds were a problem just one out of every three days, and for the entire trip only half the time, indicating that conventional wisdom didn't hold water. But considering that only four days of the roughly two months I was on the road gave me winds that actually *helped* me, the west-east route comes out on top.

From the journal:

Day 5: Sunday, May 12. 8 o'clock start. No rain when I left, but beginning at 8:40 down it came, lightly at first, then heavy at times. My rain gear kept me reasonably dry but not warm, as the temperature remained in the low 40s. From Cobleskill on NY Rte 10, it was 15 miles to US 20 at Sharon Springs, which took a bit less than two hours to cover over moderately hilly terrain. I think my legs were fatigued, for they weren't performing well and I was using the granny [lowest] gear much of the time. One blessing today—no headwind. But as I became wetter and consequently colder, I began to fantasize about a "million dollar wound" that would enable me to retire with honor and go back home.

After 35 miles on the road, I reached Richfield Springs at 11:25. When I saw a couple of motels and restaurants in the small town, I decided to call it a day. I was by then chilled to the bone. First I had lunch at a "family restaurant". Food was not good. Went next door to The Village Motel. The amiable proprietor gave me a rag to clean the bike before I brought it into the room. I put my wet clothes near a baseboard heater and had a hot shower. Bought a Sunday NY Times and spent the afternoon luxuriating in bed in the warm room and reading the paper. So-so food at a Chinese restaurant for dinner. Tomorrow I'll decide whether to go on or to rest a day here.

35 miles = 265 total

I really didn't have rain gear as such. When the weather was cold, I wore layers of clothing: a T-shirt, long-sleeve jersey, sweatshirt, and windbreaker. I wore bicycle tights over my bike shorts and covered them with a pair of semi-waterproof running pants. Some riders like fully protective waterproof clothing to keep dry, while others find that this kind of rain gear retains the body's heat, causing excessive sweating and leaving the body about as wet as it would be if not waterproofed. One way or another, you're going to get wet, so why not choose to forgo the rain gear and travel more lightly?

Perhaps on this particular day I could have kept riding longer if I had had proper rain gear. But the downpour was steady and at times quite heavy, and with the maximum temperature not getting out of the low forties, after a while I was very cold, particularly in my hands. Continuing to ride under these conditions would not have made much sense, not only because of the discomfort, but also because when the rain was heaviest, water on the road's shoulder caused me to slip and slide. In addition, it was possible that motorists could not see me until they were about on top of me.

Was I courting pneumonia? Not really. It is true that with aging the immune system loses some of its vigor, manufacturing antibodies more slowly when responding to infections. But it is also true that the trusty remedy of an active life will reduce the weakening of the immune system. Furthermore, it is well known that the cause of a cold or pneumonia is direct contact with a virus carried by someone else, not from being chilled. As it happened, in all my long-distance cycling I never once suffered from a cold or the flu and certainly did come down with a bout of pneumonia.

I was unsure how the owner of the Village Motel, a clean, well maintained one-story building of about a dozen rooms, would react to my request to take the wet mud-streaked bike into my room. He not only graciously told me to go right ahead, but also, as I noted in my journal, gave me some cleaning rags to dry and clean the bicycle. After wiping it clean, I took extra-great care not to spill any oil on the carpeted floor when I oiled the chain.

Then I walked down the main street of Richfield Springs (2000 pop. 1,255). The food of the restaurant I had chosen for lunch that afternoon and the one I went to for dinner that night was, to put it charitably, not very appetizing. One of the two was billed as a "family restaurant," which in my experience often means, "You will be much better off if you eat elsewhere."

A cross-country ride provides adventures in eating. For me, a key element in choosing motels was whether they had a café or restaurant, as some of the larger ones did, or were within walking distance of a place to eat. Only a few times were fast food joints all I could find. This was fortunate, for while they were okay for lunch, or even breakfast if nothing else was available, they could not provide the kind of meal I needed at the end of a day of riding. A positive aspect of franchises like McDonalds is that they have quality control; you generally know what you will get, although not always—for example, a barely edible burger I would have at another chain in Ohio. More important, because of the hygiene standards of the large chains, chances are that you will not fall victim to food poisoning after eating in one of their outlets, a real plus, since having to deal with stomach troubles while riding a bike in the middle of nowhere would not be fun.

As for other restaurants, the quality of those where I ate ranged from awful to superb. Two wonderful meals stick in my mind: an utterly delicious salmon steak at the Tamarisk Restaurant in Green River, Utah, and a wonderful steak dinner I had at the Buckhorn Steak and Roadhouse in Winters, California.

On average, however, the food I ate, though filling, was forgettable. For breakfast, even though pancakes are great for carbo-loading, I found them to be a risky choice: sometimes they were excellent, but about half the time, they were heavy, doughy, and unappetizing. For me, the safest bet for breakfast was eggs, bacon or sausage, potatoes, toast, juice, and coffee—lots of calories, which of course I needed.

The importance to the long-distance rider of loading up on calories at meals cannot be overstated. To keep energy levels from being depleted, carbohydrate-rich between-meal snacks are also important. They and large meals are needed to prevent what cyclists call "bonking," which occurs when the body's store of glycogen, the energy product of carbohydrates, reaches an extremely low level, resulting in an insufficient supply of fuel to the brain, as well as to muscles. When this happens, the cyclist starts to be over-fatigued and finds it hard to concentrate.

There is little if any cause to worry about gaining weight on a bicycle trek. Considering that riding all day will burn up thousands of calories, shoveling down lots of food is required to avoid losing weight. As much as I ate, I still lost several pounds on this cross-country trip. And several pounds are a lot on my 135-pound frame.

The rain came down steadily throughout the day and on into the night and the next morning, the 13th. As the day wore on it didn't let up, and I had no choice but to wait it out. I read, watched TV, and walked around town, hoping for better weather the following day, although the forecast was for more rain. And sure enough, May 14 dawned cold and showery.

From the journal:

Day 7: Tuesday, May 14. Woke up to rain showers and continued cold. Waiting for the rain to ease up, I had a superb hamburger at a hamburger stand right next to the motel—wish I'd eaten there more often. With conditions slightly improved, I got on the road at 12:20. Didn't mind the intermittent rain and the cold because I was more warmly dressed than I had been earlier, and my hands were kept warm by the fleece-lined gardening gloves I bought at Richmond Springs' hardware store at the suggestion of the motel owner after I told him my need for warm gloves. Made it north to Mohawk on NY Rte 28 in about an hour. The ride there included, after some hills, a welcome fairly steep downhill of about three miles. Rain showers fell all day long. Continued to have winds coming right at me or off my starboard bow, and progress was slow, but no hills. Riding on NY State Bicycle Route 5, now heading west I skirted Utica to its north, and just past it I stopped for a donut and hot chocolate at a convenience store. An hour after that, at Vernon, I left Rte 5 and got on NY Rte 31. As I rode on, I had a PowerBar and occasional drinks of Gatorade to help keep me going. Passed by Verona and found a motel at about 6:30. Not an easy day, but much better than Friday, Saturday, and Sunday. No further fantasizing about a way out of continuing the journey.

50 miles = 315

It was great to be back on the road, despite the less than ideal conditions. There would be some bad days ahead, but I had no more moments of mental self-flagellation for undertaking the journey. My resolve to keep going, although now and then dented or even battered early on, was never seriously in jeopardy. For one thing, discouraging occasions were more than offset by heady experiences. And in any event the thought of giving up and going home with my tail between my legs was too awful to contemplate.

I followed US Rte 20 for more than half of the ride through New York. The morning I left Richfield Springs, I rode north to Mohawk on NY 58, not returning to 20 until I reached Auburn, about 100 miles to the west. I did that because when I was planning my route, I learned from a phone call to the New York Department of Transportation that although US 20 was the most direct route for me to follow, for quite a distance to the east of Auburn the highway goes over some very steep hills. Advised to get off US 20 and go north then west to avoid that stretch of road, that's what I did.

Although the course I chose was sometimes hilly, it was for the most part a moderately undulating or level corridor northwest to Utica and Rome and from there southwest to the Finger Lakes and then west to Buffalo. In this central part of New York, I rode through land predominately given over to agriculture, dairy farms in particular. As it was too early in the spring for much planting to have begun, I passed by acres and acres of plowed and unplowed fields bare of crops. But plentiful rains had coated the countryside in a vivid, Granny-Smith-apple shade of green. I have to say, though, that however pleasant it was, until I reached Lake Erie the scenery where I rode through this part of New York wasn't very inspiring.

From the journal:

Day 8: Wednesday, May 15. Clear, windy, cool (45°). Got side-tracked immediately, missing NY Rte 31, now the bicycle route, and instead got back on NY Rte 5. This took me right into Syracuse, which I had planned to bypass to its north on Rte 31. The wind, as much as 30 mph right at my face, was awful, making the going difficult and, ultimately, exhausting. Took almost three hours, with a half-hour for lunch at Fayetteville, to get from one end of great-er Syracuse to the other. Soon afterward I had three steep climbs. Wanted to stop at 50 miles, but the only motel at the village of Elbridge was full. After another ten miles, I arrived at Auburn, where a little after 5 pm I settled on a kind of seedy motel. But the room cost only $38 and had a bed and a shower, as well as a TV for checking the Weather Channel, so who's complaining. Walked three blocks to an Applebee's for a beer and dinner of fish and chips. I'll be back on US 20 again tomorrow.

60 miles = 375 total

Construction of US 20, which runs from Boston to Oregon and is the longest highway in the United States, began in the mid-1920s, making it one of our oldest transcontinental roads. In its heyday US 20 was the most traveled east-west highway in New

York, and the area it passed through prospered accordingly. Then in the mid-1950s came the New York Thruway system, including Interstate 90, which roughly parallels US 20, running alongside it from Albany to Erie, Pennsylvania, and sucking the passenger load from it to such an extent that in the first year after I-90's construction, revenues for roadside businesses on US 20 dropped by thirty percent. As I rode along, indications of the economic downturn were plentiful along the old highway—boarded-up buildings, foundations bare of structures, and carcasses of old gas stations and motor courts, the precursors of motels. But for the cyclist, the low volume of traffic is a blessing. So too is that, despite its eclipse by I-90, US 20 is well maintained.

Driving this way three years later, I was pleasantly surprised to see that the area appeared to have taken an upturn economically, as evidenced by a lot of new commercial establishments. Certainly the general appearance of some of the towns and their environs was more pleasing to the eye than it had been when I passed by on my bike.

Day 9: Thursday, May 16. Got up early but still didn't get out of town until after 8:30. In addition to the time it takes for breakfast in places where I can get it, I'm spending too many minutes getting my stuff back into Ziploc bags and into the panniers and handlebar bag. Need to do more preparations at night and also speed things up in the morning. Had breakfast at a small local restaurant. About ten cars were parked outside, a sure sign, I thought, of good food. The menu

bragged about a secret recipe for pancakes, which to me were barely edible. For the sake of the calories I needed, I ate as much as I could.

My decision to forgo camping now made, at Geneva, 27 miles west of Auburn on US 20, I found a Mailbox, Etc. and mailed home the tent, sleeping pad, a length of rope, some bungee cords, and a few other items (e.g., extra duct tape). At 2:30 I arrived at Canandaigua [pop. 11,264]. Still somewhat fatigued from yesterday's ride and unsure how far ahead I'd have to ride before finding a motel, I decided to pack it in, even though the weather today has been the best I've encountered in the past five or six days. Got a great room at an Econo Lodge for $50. As usual I called Julie around six. The cell phone, the first I've ever had, has proven a real lifeline, and I use it to keep in touch not just with her, but also the kids and friends.

43 miles = 418 total

This separation from Julie was much more tolerable than the two lengthy separations we had during our Foreign Service life. The first, in Zanzibar in 1964, occurred because the dangers accompanying its violent revolution and immediate aftermath led to the evacuation of all Americans on the island except my boss and me. The second, much later in Sudan, came about when a supposed plot to kill the American ambassador (me) and other embassy officials caused Washington to order the departure of non-essential personnel and all family members. During those days when we were apart, we had no way to talk to each other because, except for calls to nearby Dar es Salaam on the mainland, overseas telephone service from Zanzibar was next to non-existent. And although the overseas service did function in Sudan, I never managed to get a call through to Mexico City, where she had gone to be with her family while awaiting word from Washington that she and Brian could return. In view of that history, it was especially nice now to have the cell phone for evening conversations with her.

It would soon turn cold again, but on the day I rode from Auburn to Canandaigua the maximum temperature rose to 70° under a partly cloudy sky. Approaching Canandaigua from the south, I passed through the western edge of the town, which overlooks Lake Canandaigua. After I'd settled in at a motel, I read in a bookstore in town that the name Canandaigua is derived from an Iroquois word meaning "the chosen spot." That is apt, given the beautiful view of the lake from the town. This day the lake was ruffled by the wind and tinted silver and blue by sun and sky, and as I rode up a hill toward the town, I stopped for a while to admire the scene.

From the journal:

Day 10: Friday, May 17. Chilly, about 40° when I left Canandaigua at 9:30, late because I'd overslept. Headwind recurred but not very strong, maybe ten mph. Encountered some hills and it seemed that, overall, there was a gradual increase in altitude for many miles. [Not so. I later found that the towns west of Canandaigua all the way to Buffalo were actually slightly lower than Canandaigua in elevation.] At Avon I took a wrong turn that took me off US 20 and onto NY Rte 5 again. Five miles later, at Le Roy, the birthplace of Jell-O and home of the Jell-O Museum, I found a road back to US 20 and continued west. By this time I'd ridden about 50 miles. Le Roy and Avon were pleasant-appearing towns, but except for Alden, all the other towns along US 20 this day were unprepossessing. Countryside was nice though—farms, many of them dairy farms, for miles and miles.

Not long after I'd gotten back on US 20, I stopped at a gas station to get advice on a place to stay. Was told I would find a motel in Alden, 20 miles down the road. But all that Alden had to offer were two unattractive motels with no nearby place to eat. I'd gone about 70 miles at this point. Got directions to divert off of US 20 about 15 miles farther on and ride to a commercial area, where I'd find hotels and motels. Finally, at about 8:30, as it was getting dark, 11 hours after leaving Canandaigua I arrived at a Sheraton Hotel. I got a room, had a beer, and ate dinner. Am I tired? Yep, but also pleased about the length of today's ride. I'm four miles east of Buffalo.

90 miles = 508 total

"Weather Underground" (www.wunderground.com) is the

website I chose to obtain, after the fact, data such as wind veloci-ties and temperatures for the dates at the locations where I rode. Its "History and Almanac" section has information about cities and towns or nearby weather reporting stations for any day going back to 1948. To get the elevation and other geographical data of places I passed through on the trip I drew on information from the U.S. Geological Survey's website, geonames.usgs.gov.

Eleven and a half hours to ride 90 miles is pretty slow going. Hills and a headwind largely accounted for the 7.8 mph average. In ad-dition, I lost time when I took the wrong turn at Avon and again when I had to seek directions at Alden. Not only that, I added another 40 minutes to the day's ride when I didn't stop at the Sheraton, thinking that since it was a somewhat expensive hotel I'd not be able to take my bike into my room. The more modest hotel I came to farther down the road was full, so I decided go back and try the Sheraton, where to my surprise I found that they were more than willing to let me bring the bike into the hotel and up to my room.

The failure to find a decent place to stay in Alden illustrated the risk of not being sure what accommodations would be avail-able at the end of the day. Nevertheless, not once on the trip was I unable to find a motel or hotel. The worst that happened was that now and then to be sure to get a motel room, I ended a day's ride earlier that I preferred.

I was sorely tempted to have a look at the Jell-O Museum at

Le Roy. Like many other red-blooded Americans, at least of my generation, Jell-O was a favorite dessert when I was a little kid, especially when it had some whipped cream on top. But at Le Roy and other points along the way, in favor of satisfying an inner compulsion to get to San Francisco in as short a time as I could, I passed up most sightseeing opportunities, especially those that would involve a detour. More important, summer was approaching, and the earlier I got to the long, hot expanses of roads in Utah and Nevada, the better.

One important goal of a newcomer to long-distance cycling is a "century," the term for a 100-mile ride in a day. The 90 miles I rode this day under less than optimal conditions indicated that I ought to be able to get my century at some point in the journey. As it was, I was pleased to have gone as far as I did and also to be within a day of Lake Erie. At the hotel bar before I went to the dining room that night, I hoisted a couple of beers, one to celebrate the 90-mile ride and another because I'd passed the 500-mile mark today.

I don't want to give an impression that I had an alcoholic or near-alcoholic urge for beer at the end of each day. It's just that I like its taste, unlike soft drinks it doesn't dull one's appetite for food, and—in strict moderation—beer is a healthier drink than the sugary alternatives. At least that's how I look at it, while knowing that both beverages have their downsides and that water is the healthiest drink of all. But, c'mon, at the end of a physically demanding hot day during which I drink lots of water, I'm supposed to want more of the same?

From the journal:

Day 11: Saturday, May 18. Slept in until 7:15. Yesterday's long ride had tired me out. Because it was a chilly 39° and rainy, I delayed starting until 10:15. As I was about to leave the Sheraton's driveway, a small truck approached on the road I was about to enter. It was flashing its emergency lights instead of a turn indictor, and having no idea what the driver was going to do, I braked hard but so clumsily that I couldn't release my shoe cleats quickly and down I went. It was a hard fall, but no damage was done to the bike or to me.

During the day, the temperature never rose above 45°. However, finally for a change there was no wind, and I made good time. For 33 miles there was no sign of a restaurant, or of much else. The depressing effects that the nearby interstate highway I-90 has had on Rte 20's roadside businesses was apparent yesterday, when I found it impossible to find a motel until I almost reached Buffalo. I encountered a similar scarcity again today. Thus when I came across a Ramada Inn at Dunkirk [pop. 13,131] at 3:00, I asked someone whether there were any motels within 20 or so miles down the road. Told there weren't any, I checked in. At $80, my room is pricey, but the restaurant has good food and affords a great view of Lake Erie.

47 miles = 555 total

The staff at the Ramada Inn was as pleasant as could be. A couple of them were Mexicans, and as I often do when I run into people from Mexico or Central or South America, I spoke Spanish with them. I had an intensive course in conversational Spanish when I entered the Foreign Service in 1960 and greatly improved my ability to speak and understand the language when I went to my first post, the American Embassy in Mexico. It didn't hurt that the Mexican girl I got acquainted with, courted, and married seven months after I arrived in Mexico City spoke no English when we met.

The two Mexicans at the motel had emigrated from Mexico several years earlier, and they spoke passable English, but responded in Spanish when I spoke it. As often happens when I converse with Spanish speakers, they wanted to know where and how I had learned their language. Because some of the Latinos I have met in this country might not be legal immigrants, if I have any doubt about their status, I don't ask questions about how they had come to live where they were working. By nature curious about people's backgrounds, I have no such compunctions when talking to Anglo waitresses or waiters. Frequently the young among them are students; my waitress at dinner that night was enrolled at nearby State University of New York at Fredonia. The young woman who served me at breakfast the following morning told me she was a single mother of a little girl.

I read Barbara Ehrenrich's *Nickel and Dimed* not long after the book was published in 2001. In it she describes how she attempted to eke out a living while working as a waitress, hotel maid, house cleaner, nursing home aide, and Wal-Mart associate. It is a jarring account of the plight of America's working poor, who struggle to survive on what they earn in their low-paying, often physically exhausting, jobs. Before reading *Nickel and Dimed,* I thought I was a reasonably generous tipper, especially after one of my daughters told me of her experiences when she spent a summer working as a waitress in a nightclub in Washington, DC. But Ehrenrich's account convinced me to tip even higher and never, never, ever to forget to leave some money for the hotel maid who would clean my room after I left.

Day 12: Sunday, May 19. Slept in until 7 again. It didn't freeze last night—low temperature 37°. Weather Channel predicts a high of 45 today, and wind will not be a problem (10 mph from the north). I am now applying sunscreen liberally. Had just been putting some dabs here and there on my face, not including the space between nose and upper lip. Result was sunburn.

Couldn't ask for better weather: sunny, cool, clear blue sky flecked with scattered cumulus clouds inland from the lake, and as predicted, only a light breeze from my right. Beautiful vistas today: Lake Erie a deep blue-green, occasional golf courses, attractive lakeside houses and cottages, creeks flowing down to the lake, great swaths of verdant grass and, after mile 20, numerous small vineyards. The road, Pennsylvania Rte 5, was little trafficked this Sunday morning and afternoon. On a country road such as this, when the traffic is extremely light, I find it okay to leave the shoulder and ride on the roadway. But when I spy a car coming toward me, I get back on the shoulder, even if I don't think there are any cars behind me. This is only prudent, for the noise of the approaching vehicle could mask the sound of one or more approaching from behind.

Two days ago I lost my map of the area between Buffalo and Erie,

Pennsylvania. My guess that today's ride to Erie would be from 30-35 miles was incorrect; the distance actually was 47 miles. After a hamburger for lunch, I crossed into Pennsylvania at 1:30. The quality of the roadway and, especially, the shoulder improved markedly when I left New York. Curiously, there was an unusually large number of dead birds along the road. Now I passed vineyards of greater acreage than those I had seen in New York. Erie, at least the parts I rode through, was a handsome city, with prosperous-looking residential areas. After I stopped to ask a young woman for directions, we had a conversation. A college student, she, like almost all the people I have talked to on this trip, was friendly and seemed genuinely interested to know what I'm doing. At about 4:45 I found a motel—a tiny, 1930s-vintage place, with an Italian deli nearby. Cheese pizza and ice cream for supper.

57 miles = 612 total

Because of the cool-to-cold weather and sometimes overcast skies, I hadn't given much thought to sunscreen. For a couple of days, I thought the burning sensation on parts of my face was windburn. This was foolish of me because I have know for many years that unless cloud cover is thick, it does not give protection against the sun's ultra-violet rays, which can damage exposed skin. Once I realized what accounted for the burn, I took care to liberally apply sunscreen before setting out each day and generally remembered to put on some more after I had been riding for several hours.

Skin is going to wrinkle with aging, a natural process that

begins in the mid-20s, though its effects are usually not visible until years later. In time the skin becomes thinner and also begins to sag and lose its ability to go back into place after being stretched. Overexposure to the sun's ultraviolet rays speeds up and intensifies the process, causing excessive wrinkling because of a more than normal breakdown of the components of the mid-layer of the skin. Of much more concern than loose skin and wrinkling is the development of pre-cancerous and cancerous damage from the ultra-violet rays—pre-cancerous actinic keretoses, cancerous basal-cell and squamous-cell carcinomas, and the dreaded melanoma.

The best preventive measure against wrinkling and serious skin damage is to stay out of the sun. So those who want to keep their skin as youthful-looking as possible should not consider long-distance bicycle trips. Even with the application of a sunscreen, riding a bike for hours at a time is bound to have a detrimental effect on the skin. People who enjoy the physical and psychic benefits of outdoor activities, including bicycling, are not likely to be turned off by the prospect of some additional wrinkling. Certainly I wasn't. Nevertheless, slathering exposed skin areas with a sunscreen having an SPF rating of at least 30 is necessary to forestall burning and to reduce the chances of developing serious skin damage.

The foundation for skin damage is laid long before we get old, with the result that many elderly folks, like me, are living examples of the long-term effects of over-exposure to the sun's rays when we were young and, in those days, ignorant of the harm we were inflicting on ourselves. People of a certain age will remember applying baby oil while baking in the sun, a sure way to cook the skin.

Short of resorting to plastic or laser surgery, we can't do away with wrinkles and loose skin and are pretty much stuck with "liver spots," as the brownish blemishes of the skin are called. These, which vary in size and usually appear on the face, hands, shoulders, and arms, have nothing to do with the liver and everything to do with the sun. Unlike cancerous or pre-cancerous blemishes, the age spots are benign, but they certainly do look like hell.

Sun exposure is an important source of vitamin D and should not be avoided entirely. But old people should realize that our aged, thinner skin is very vulnerable to harmful reactions to sunshine. Even more so than younger people, the elderly should apply sunscreen, wear a hat and long sleeves, use sunglasses that block ultra-violet rays, avoid like the plague tanning booths and sunlamps, and keep a close eye out for changing moles and new growths.

CHAPTER 6

The Midwest

Living as you do in New York, the navel of the universe, it is easy to confuse the Midwest and the South.

John Fleischman

Well, I was born and raised in the Midwest, in Indiana specifically, and my childhood was full of weekend movies, you know, the Saturday and Sunday popcorn movies.

Sydney Pollack

From the journal:

Day 13: Monday, May 20. On the road at 8:45. Temp. 30°, skies partly cloudy, not much wind, another good day for cycling. Before leaving the motel, I ate a half slice of cold pizza (couldn't abide any more than that) and half an energy bar. Started looking for a place to eat, but didn't come across one until I'd gone 23 miles. By then Rte 5 had merged with US Rte 20. Crossed into Ohio at about 10:30. As soon as I was in Ohio the road quality deteriorated. No shoulder to speak of, the highway itself pot-holed and very cracked. Found a diner in Conneaut at 10:45. Good pancakes. Learned that there was a bicycle shop in Ashtabula, 12 miles away. The roadway improved as I neared Ashtabula, and traffic became fairly heavy. At the bike shop I had the gearshift fixed (cable was loose and I couldn't shift onto the largest of the front rings). The shop's owner gave me advice on a better route south than the one I had tentatively chosen. Kept going southwest to Geneva—eight miles from Ashtabula—where I turned south. Three miles later, I checked into a Howard Johnson, the last motel for many miles. The bar/grille across the street was closed, so I ended up at a fast food joint, where I had the worst hamburger ever.

48 miles = 660 total

That night, when I wrote my journal entry for the day's ride I didn't mention a near disaster in Ashtabula. As I rode away from the bike shop and got back on US 20, I heard a plop and, looking back, saw my wallet in the middle of the road. Had I lost it, I would have been in deep trouble—*sans* credit cards, ID and cash. I suppose Julie could have wired me some money to tide me over, but I really needed a credit card and would have been stuck in Ashtabula until a replacement arrived. One lesson learned: I took my spare credit card out of my wallet and kept it in a saddlebag.

I would have more episodes of potentially calamitous forgetfulness on the journey.

From the journal:

Day 14: Tuesday, May 21. Before starting yesterday, I adjusted the saddle to a less-elevated angle to see if it would be more comfortable. It wasn't. I kept sliding forward and had to use hand and arm strength to counter the forward slide. This morning I readjusted the saddle, and that worked out for the better. Continental breakfast at the Howard Johnson was coffee and a choice of pastries; I ate two chocolate éclairs. Left the motel at 8:20 on Ohio Rte 534 heading due south and began looking for a place to eat. Rode through farm country and saw no restaurants or even a convenience store until, 33 miles later, I reached Windham and found a small restaurant. After eating, I got on Ohio Rte 5, which took me west again. Another 30 miles or so I came across a strip mall at Rootstown that had a restaurant and supermarket. Had a BLT and a long, pleasant conversation with an old guy (look who's talking) who was interested in what I was doing and told me about some of his WWII adventures. I had missed Ravenna, where I'd planned to look for a place to stay. Ohio Rte 5 bypassed Ravenna, and seeing no sign showing how to get to the town, I ended up in Rootstown instead. My lunch companion there had given me great directions that took me on a county road not shown on my map and got me to US 43 and on to Brimfield, which was very close to Akron. There were some motels close by, adjoining I-76, and I chose a Ramada Inn. Had an early evening beer and convivial conversation with bar denizens, who seemed impressed with what I was doing. Weather was good again today—temp 32° at the start and 49° at the end. Wind was not a problem.

71 miles = 731 total

I took some pains to ensure as well as I could that my bike would not be stolen. If that happened, obviously I would be up a creek without any means to keep going. Not only would I not have a bicycle, I would also have lost everything in my saddlebags (but not the handlebar bag; I always took it with me when I stopped to eat). At eating places I either tethered the bike with my cable lock to an immovable fixture or, if there was none, parked it where I could keep an eye on it while I ate. Until this day, I never had a problem. After lunch I trundled the bike over to the supermarket in the strip mall. Not finding anything at the store that I could use for securing the bike with the lock, I looked around and saw an alternative—an extra-long line of shopping carts in the store's parking lot. I figured it wasn't going anywhere and fastened the cable lock to a cart in the middle of the pack. I was in the store for just a few minutes. When I came out I was horrified to see that the carts and my bike had disappeared. But whatever power it is that sometimes forgives incompetency saved me again, for there, as I got closer, I spied my trusty Cannondale lying on the ground undamaged and with all its appurtenances, except the cable lock. I had attached the lock to the cart but, incredibly, failed to put it around the bike frame. Somewhere in Rootstown a shopping cart may still be adorned with a red and black cable lock.

From the journal:

Day 15: Wednesday, May 22. Today, according to the Weather Channel, has been the last day of a record cold spell for this part of the country. It was 31° when I got up and I'd say about 35° when I left at 8:20. After a couple of hours, and for the first time since I left New Hampshire, I took off my sweatshirt. [The maximum temperature for the area that day was 71°.] Because I had a continental breakfast at the motel, I didn't have to look for a restaurant on the road. Went south five miles to Ohio Rte 224 then west to Barberton. The Akron suburban traffic was heavy, and after taking a wrong turn I found myself headed for a major artery into the city. Got off it, obtained directions for backstreets to Ohio 585, and had lunch at a diner when I reached it.

Rte 585 was a trial. Shoulders were only six inches to a foot, fairly heavy traffic, lots of trucks. I wouldn't recommend this route. Both before I got to Barberton and along 585, I encountered some steep hills. By the time I got to Wooster [pop. 24,811], 24 miles later, I was ready to call it a day and decided to look for a motel or hotel. Found one several blocks away. Clearly, the length of my rides is going to continue to be governed to a large extent by the availability of a place to stay. I could have gone farther today but would have had to ride as much as another 43 miles before finding a motel, which would have really wrung me out, given today's headwind and the hills that I'm sure lie ahead.

52 miles = 783 total

In the late fall of 2001, after I bought the bicycle, began learning to ride, and started to build up my endurance, I went out only on days when the temperature was above 50°. The forward movement of the bicycle increases wind-chill, and I didn't like the cold. But now, with temperatures close to or below freezing in the early morning, I had no choice. Had I waited for 50° temperatures, I might still have been in New Hampshire. What I discovered was that riding in the lower temperatures, as long as I was dressed warmly enough, was not bad at all. In fact, pedaling along in cold or cool mornings on days when the wind had decided to spare me was invigorating, a real joy. Days like those and other cycling pleasures, such as coasting downhill, talking to people, seeing new places, feasting on beautiful scenery, knowing I did well in completing a long or difficult ride, and having a good meal and a comfortable bed at night more than made up for the times when wind and hills had their way with me.

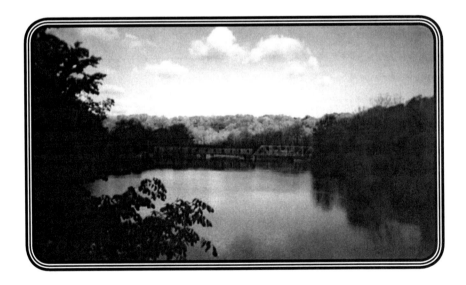

Covered bridge along the road to Wooster

Day 16: Thursday, May 23. US 3 out of Wooster *presented the same absence of decent road shoulders for miles, but after about three hours they widened. The highway runs southwest, and today's 15 mph wind was from, guess what, the southwest! All day long, as I passed through the hills of this part of Ohio, I struggled with the sometimes very steep inclines. The hills and wind took the starch out of me, and a couple of times I had to stop to rest. Even though I only went 42 miles today, I believe this has been the most physically tiring day I've had thus far. I am zonked. Arrived in Mount Vernon [pop. 15,256] a little after 3:00 and stopped at a hotel right in the center of this small town.*

42 miles = 825 total

I didn't leave Wooster until 8:30. With a half hour for lunch, I was on the bike for six hours. The average speed of seven mph indicates the slow going imposed by wind and hills and also why the short ride of 42 miles tired me out. Twelve years have gone by since I wrote my journal, and I'm not sure why the entry for the Wooster to Mt. Vernon ride is so brief and short on details. But maybe it was because I was short on energy that night.

A topographical map shows that much of the northeastern and southeastern parts of central Ohio are dominated by bedrock hills. This certainly applied to my route, as I rode southwest from Barberton through Wooster to Mount Vernon. I had read an account by a transcontinental bike rider who said the eastern Ohio hills were an unexpectedly tough part of his journey. Knowing that, I still wasn't prepared for the amount of steep hills I would have to climb. They would not have been nearly as tiring had it not been for the vexatious headwinds along the way.

The work I had done to climb the Appalachians in Vermont and my battles with hills here in Ohio as well as other places along my way required a fair amount of muscle strength. One of the most obvious effects of aging is that muscle strength declines. This happens because beginning at about age 30 or 35, muscle mass gradually decreases as the number and size of muscle fibers goes down. The loss of muscle mass affects larger muscle groups, thigh and calf muscles for example, much more than smaller ones. Therefore, by age 40 most professional athletes can no longer compete, while musicians, pianists for example, perform skillfully well into old age.

Like the decrease of bone mass, the reduction of muscle mass is a natural process, but the rate of decline varies with one's lifestyle and level of fitness. It should come as no surprise that physical inactivity accelerates muscle mass loss whereas regular exercise can significantly offset the loss and its accompanying reduction in strength.

However, note that the operative word is "offset", not halt. No matter what you do for exercise, as you get up in years you are going to have lower muscle tone, as lean muscle tissue decreases and more fat is deposited into muscles. Simply put, you will not be as strong as when you were younger. If you are a runner, for example, regardless of how much you train, after a certain age the passage of years will reduce speed and endurance. But regular physical activity will make you stronger than you otherwise would be and allow you to enjoy life much more fully.

On the coming day, shortly after leaving Mt. Vernon I would put behind me the worst hills I would encounter for another 1,400 miles. Not that there wouldn't be some tough riding between there and the Rocky Mountains; if nothing else, headwinds would ensure that. And I'd have to overcome some muscle fatigue—caused by a failure to train hard enough and long enough before setting out, or by occasional dehydration, or perhaps by pushing my age-related limits a bit too much too soon. All three factors probably were involved. Later I would get stronger, to an extent that sometimes surprised me.

From the journal:

Day 17: Friday, May 24. Started later than I wanted and by the time I found a convenience store that had bananas and another store that sold Gatorade, it was almost 9 o'clock. Headed due west on Ohio Rte 229. Expecting more of the same as yesterday, lots of steep climbs, I was pleasantly surprised that after five miles of only a few inclines, the terrain leveled off. Hooray! A 10-15 mph headwind slowed me down and continued to do so after I turned southwest on Ohio 42 at Ashley, 26 miles from Mt. Vernon. But the wind began to diminish and I made good time to Delaware, a larger town than the others I passed through today, and had a roast beef sandwich for lunch. The restaurant was filled with overweight people, most of them smoking cigarettes and all of them eating big platefuls of carbo-loaded food.

Although, as far as I know, the incidence of cigarette smoking in the states I passed through was the same or close to the same as in New Hampshire, it seemed higher to me, perhaps because I was spending time in bars or taverns for a post-ride beer and almost never frequented them at home. Also, in New Hampshire Julie and I dined out at smoke-free restaurants, while most of the places where I ate in the smaller towns on my trip did not have a no-smoking area, much less a ban on smoking. (I imagine that has changed by now.)

It is depressing that cigarette smoking continues to be the leading preventable cause of premature death in the United States. And when smokers are overweight they are begging for severe health problems. But it's no mystery why, even after so much publicity about the dangers of smoking and of obesity, so many overweight Americans smoke: Cigarette smoking is so addictive that quitting is extremely difficult and, as the millions of diet books published in this country indicate and medical research confirms, shedding pounds also is far from an easy proposition.

Again I am impelled to beat the drum for exercise, in this instance because exercise can help people kick the smoking habit and also to lose weight. I smoked for almost 40 years until, in my 50s, I trained to run a marathon. Becoming smoke-free is important to consider seriously if you want not only to prolong your life, but also to improve your health in the process. Besides, you smell—and I am referring to both the transitive and the intransitive verb—much better.

Back to journal entry for May 24, day 17:

A mile or so after riding out of Delaware, I realized I was on the wrong road, returned to town, and got directions for Marysville, about 20 miles away on Rte 36. Ran into rain showers a couple of times, but they didn't last long, and I made it to Marysville [pop. 22,094] at about 4. Owing to some bad directions from several people, 20 minutes passed before I talked to a man who knew the area well and set me straight on where I'd find accommodations. Checked into a Day's Inn. For over half my ride today the road's shoulder was from zero to a few inches wide. Fortunately the traffic was not heavy. Once, though, a few miles out of Mount Vernon, while I was going up a hill four big trucks, one after the other, came at me from the other direction at a fast clip. The wind they generated almost knocked me off the road.

Know I'm pushing it a bit too hard. I've been fatigued at the end of the ride these past three days and my quadriceps ache. Nevertheless, I'm pretty sure that the land will be flatter and I'll have easier riding in Indiana and Illinois, I'm intent on getting out of Ohio as soon as I can.

57 miles = 882

The Midwest is variously defined as a geographical, cultural and political region of the United States, but it lacks distinct boundaries. Of the states I would be crossing, Ohio, Indiana, Illinois, Missouri and Kansas are considered Midwestern, although to some geographers Ohio is in the East rather than the Midwest. When I rode into Ohio from Pennsylvania I had no sense of moving into a different region. But as I got farther west it seemed to me that the character of the towns, countryside, and people I encountered took on a Midwestern cast. I can't really define this, but perhaps my feeling is akin to what Supreme Court Justice Potter Stewart said about pornography—you know it when you see it.

After I left the hillier eastern part of Ohio and until I reached Kansas, the Midwestern terrain I passed through consisted of gently rolling hills and some welcome level stretches. I learned later that the flat interruptions of the rolling landscape are where glacial ice or small lakes once stood thousands of years ago. The area between the geologically ancient Alleghenies and the middle-aged Rocky Mountains has, except for the Black Hills of South Dakota, a mainly low topographical profile. When I checked the elevations of the towns on my route, I found that, from Bennington, Vermont, until I got to Kansas, the elevation fluctuated between about 500 and 1,000 feet, with a high at Mt. Vernon, Ohio, of 1,020 feet and a low of 491 feet at Hannibal, Missouri.

There is nothing majestic about Midwestern scenery, but there is much that is pleasant. A great proportion of the country I passed through was farmland, as would be expected in the Midwest. However, it was interspersed with wooded hills, meadows, meandering creeks, slowly flowing rivers, and ponds or lakes.

Across the country, I passed through or by a few large cities, a fair number of small to mid-size cities, and many small towns. There's no denying that, although there are many exceptions, most American towns are not works of beauty, to put it kindly. Some of those I saw in the Midwest had attractive features, such as graceful late nineteenth or early twentieth century Victorian houses along quiet streets lined with shade trees. But the downtowns generally had little to commend them. As was true in most of the rest of the country, Midwestern towns were not built with esthetics in mind when they sprang up in the nineteenth century. In 1900 a French visitor referred to the hasty and utilitarian construction of American towns. In 1927, the iconoclastic critic H.L. Mencken put it more bluntly. Comparing European and American towns, he said: "There is scarcely an ugly village on the whole Continent. The peasants, however poor, somehow manage to make themselves graceful and charming habitations, even in Spain. But in the American village and small town the pull is always toward ugliness...."[8] Mencken may have been too unsparing in his judgment, and in any case he neglected to mention that Europe had its share of squalid villages.

In the twentieth century the arrival and vast increase in numbers of automobiles in America scarred towns and cities with car lots, gas stations, garages, and other facilities for cars. And then, after World War II, came the introduction of featureless housing subdivisions, ugly strip malls, big box stores, and fast-food franchises, all adding to the unattractive homogenization of a great many American towns and cities.

8   "The Libido of the Ugly," *Prejudices, Sixth Series* (New York: Harper, 1927).

From the journal:

Day 18: Saturday, May 25. Got underway at 8:25. Would have left earlier but waited until a heavy rain shower passed. My map showed that the only way out of town heading west would be on the Ohio Rte 4 by-pass, on which US Rte 36 merged. When I got there I found that bicycles are prohibited. So I rode back into town and got directions. I was told that I could get to US 36 by way of Milford Avenue to a county road southwest of Milford Center. It was a good road, no traffic to speak of, and under an overcast sky and in some light fog I made it to Milford Center in about an hour. A few miles afterward, I came to US 36, no longer merged with the Rte 4 by-pass. It took me on a more westerly course for, first, Urbana, and then Piqua (pronounced Pick-way), population about 20,000. There I got a room at a Comfort Inn located in a mall. The terrain today was gently undulating with no steep hills, which was lucky for me because my legs became fatigued from coping with a persistent headwind that rose to 15 mph in the afternoon.

58 miles = 940 total

Day 19: Sunday, May 26. It was good I arrived in Piqua when I did yesterday afternoon. Later in the day a violent thunderstorm with heavy rain and strong winds rolled through. Forgot to mention that for well over half the trip yesterday the roads had no shoulders. That wasn't so today, at least not until I got to Indiana. This morning, by the time I'd made a stop at a convenience store, ridden from the east end of Piqua to the other end of town, got lost, and got directions, it was 9:30 am. US 36 west from Piqua had a shoulder of as much as two feet in width much of the time. No significant wind at all today. Traveling over the flat countryside, I made it to Greenville shortly before 11:30, averaging 12 mph. After breakfast/lunch there, I took Ohio Rte 502 to the Indiana line, which I crossed at 12:40. About a mile later I turned south on Indiana Rte 227. No shoulder, but no problem, since there was hardly any traffic until I got close to Richmond [pop. 39,124].

In Richmond at 3 pm, I called Mike Nixon, a cross-country cyclist whose name I'd found on the Internet and with whom I'd exchanged emails when I was planning my trip. He'd invited me to stay at his house when I came through Richmond. Mike, a genial young man, picked me up, took me and the bike to his home, where I showered and changed clothes. We drove to a friend's house, where I met Mike's family and his friends who had gathered for a Memorial Day barbecue. I enjoyed the food, the company, and the chance to rest for the remainder of the day.

57 miles = 997 total

Although, as I noted earlier, I did not use the Internet to search for information about lodgings and bike shops, in seeking advice about roads, I had exchanged emails with a number of people. Along with giving me helpful information, some of my correspondents invited me to stay in their homes if I came their way. Unfortunately, it so happened that except for Mike Nixon's, all the invitations were for places that were not on or close to my eventual route. No matter, the offers, which showed goodwill to a stranger, were what counted.

Mike had ridden most of the way from Los Angeles to Washington, DC, a few years earlier and gave me some good advice. Justifiably proud of his family's tool and die manufacturing business, after the barbeque he gave me a tour of the building housing the machinery. The next day, he rode with me to Indianapolis on US 40. The sky was clear and there was hardly any wind. Conversing as we rode, we made good time by my standard—the first 26 miles in two hours—as Mike rode at a leisurely pace on his road bike to stay with me. After 57 miles we stopped and waited for Mike's lovely wife, Lisa, and their two little girls to arrive in the Nixons' car. When they did, we put the bikes on the car and drove to the Bicycle Garage—the biggest bicycle shop I have ever seen—where I bought a cable lock to replace the one I lost six days earlier at the supermarket in Rootstown. Then we went to a Mexican restaurant for lunch, after which they drove me to the western part of Indianapolis and dropped me off near US 36, where I rode to a motel. Although I had not been bothered by the general solitude of my journey, the time I spent with Mike and his family and friends was an enjoyable change of pace.

The 57 miles we rode from Richmond into Indianapolis brought my total mileage to 1,054.

From the journal:

Day 21: Tuesday, May 28. Made an earlier start at 7:10. With the days getting hotter, I'm going to need to get rolling as early as possible. Temperature this morning was 65° and rose to 80°. At this point, US Rte 36 was a four-lane divided highway with lots of traffic but also having a wide, smooth shoulder.

For about 20 miles the road was flat to Danville, where it became two lanes, the shoulder disappeared, and the traffic became relatively light. After Danville, I encountered hills, one long but not too steep, and three or four not as long but so steep that I had to shift to the lowest gear. I had had a complimentary continental breakfast at the motel. The cereal and pastries weren't enough to sustain me for the morning, but there was no place to eat along the highway. Made do with "energy gel", a banana, and Gatorade. Finally, after 43 miles from my start, I came to a restaurant in the vicinity of Raccoon Lake. Had a late breakfast of eggs, bacon, toast, hash browns and milk. Continuing on US 36, I reached Rockville [pop. 2,765] less than an hour later and, after scouting out the two motels I located, I chose the one close to Weber's Kountry Kitchen, for the other had nothing but fast-food places within walking distance.

After showering and washing my clothes, I walked into town. I've concluded that I really don't need my khaki trousers, since I'll most likely wear shorts from here on out and if I need long pants, I can use my rain pants. Nor do I think I'll need the sleeping bag. So, in keeping with my aim to get rid of every unnecessary pound of weight, I took the sleeping bag and trousers to the post office and mailed them home. Ate two ice cream bars and returned to the motel, whose rate, $35, tax included, is the lowest so far.

I'm a bit worried that the sometimes loud noise of traffic is going to damage my hearing. Tomorrow I'll see whether the earplugs I bought will be helpful. The muscle soreness I've been experiencing has, until now, been confined to my quadriceps, but when I got off the bike today and began walking around, both calves were sore.

57 miles = 1,111 Total

The earplugs didn't pan out. They weren't a good idea in the first place, in that if effective they might keep me from hearing cars or trucks coming up from behind. But in fact they did not quell enough noise to warrant their use.

Like the energy bars I had been eating, the energy gel I had this morning claimed to provide quick energy. Many people swear by the hyped benefits of energy boosters. The bars, particularly those consisting mainly of carbohydrates, are a good source of energy, but I found them to be dubious value as a source of *quick* energy, or as some advertising would make you believe, a "burst" of a great gob of energy.

After they were first marketed in a big way about 30 years ago with the invention of the PowerBar, energy bars quickly gained popularity. A proliferation of different brands was accompanied by aggressive, sometimes over-the-top advertising. It wasn't long before energy bars went out of favor, largely because, with high-fructose corn syrup as a main ingredient, many brands were simply candy bars in disguise. In time and with more defensible contents they regained a favorable reputation with consumers, even though it is questionable that they are more effective than other sources of carbohydrate-sourced calories in aiding the performance of endurance athletes. But I suppose a "healthy" energy bar with good ingredients was better for me nutritionally than a candy bar.

From the journal:

Day 22: Wednesday, May 29. Evidently the muscle soreness was a sign of fatigue, for today what should have been an easy ride was difficult. Because of bad planning last night, all I had to fortify me when I started out from Rockville at 6:15 were three Oreo cookies and a cup of coffee. Forecast was for another day like yesterday—warm and humid with a chance of showers. The sky was leaden all morning, but no rain fell. I kept going due west on US 36. The wind was generally light from the southwest but nonetheless enough to slow me down a little. The route was level all the way to Montezuma (where did it get that name?) ten miles away, where I had a sandwich for breakfast at a coffee and sandwich shop, the only food source available. Ran into small hills afterward for a few miles, then flat terrain for the rest of the day. Crossed the Wabash River, and five miles afterward entered Illinois at 7:45.

Farther down the road, at 10:30 I found a restaurant and had a good breakfast. As the morning wore on, my legs weakened to the point that, in addition to stopping briefly to stand for a couple of minutes, I dismounted twice and sat down by the roadside to rest. At 1 pm I reached Tuscola, a town, according to a road sign, of 4,500 inhabitants where I got a room at an Amerhost Inn. After cleaning my riding clothes and myself, I went across the highway for a couple

*of hamburgers at a McDonald's. Fatigue and sore calves tell me I
should rest here tomorrow, but I'll wait until the morning to decide.*

59 miles = 1170 total

Over the years I have been to all 50 US states and have found the
origin of place names fascinating. Why are a number of towns in
some states named Montezuma, for example? Post-ride googling
revealed that eight states have Montezumas—New York, Ohio,
Illinois, Indiana, Iowa, Kansas, Colorado, and New Mexico. I
could find no explanation for why the early residents of these
towns chose the name of an Aztec emperor. Ohio's website says it
best: "The origin of the town's name remains a mystery."

The sources of American place names are many and varied,
and my trip would take me to some colorful examples. In upstate
New York I passed through or by Troy, Utica, Rome, and Syracuse,
all named during a late eighteenth-century classical revival in the
United States. Later on I passed through Mesopotamia, Ohio,
and Hannibal, Missouri. Piqua, Ohio, was a typical example of
an English language approximation of an Indian word, in this instance Pickawillany, which was shortened to Piqua. Place names
borrowed from Indian words have been bestowed on towns and
cities in every state. More than half of state names have Indian
origins. On my route, Topeka (said to be a Kaw word meaning
"to dig good potatoes"), Kansas (Sioux word for "south wind people"), is one of three instances in which both the name of the state
and its capital are of Indian origin. I rode by Cotopaxi, Colorado,

named by the town's founder, who had mined in South America and thought the mountains of the area were similar to Mount Cotopaxi, a volcano in Ecuador. Battle Mountain, Nevada, supposedly—no one knows for sure—got its name from a hostile encounter between whites and Indians, probably won by the whites, for, as George R. Stewart noted, if the whites won, it was a battle; if they lost, it was a massacre.[9]

From the journal:

Day 23: Thursday, May 30. Had cramps in my calf muscles last night. Spent the day holed up in my motel room in Tuscola, resting and trying to get the kinks out of my legs. Applied moist heat with a wet towel and took a hot bath three times. McDonalds was the only restaurant within easy walking distance, so I had to rely on it for all three meals today. This evening the worst of the leg soreness is gone, and I plan to ride tomorrow.

The muscle cramps in Illinois were to a large extent a result of dehydration, which could also have contributed to my fatigue. The weather was getting much warmer, and I wasn't drinking enough to replace the fluid I was losing. One book on long-distance cycling states that you should drink no less than 20 ounces

---

9   *Names on the Land* (New York: Random House, 1945) 252.

of fluid per hour while riding on a hot day. Perhaps that is so, but like a lot of across-the-board advice, that figure may not apply to everyone. Speaking for myself, I would find it a pain to have to glug down five ounces or more of water or sports drink every 15 minutes and, furthermore, I don't believe that I need *that* much. Nonetheless, I was not drinking enough and was paying a price. Between Illinois and Colorado I would experience muscle cramps a few more times, but finally, after consciously increasing my fluid intake, I had no further problems with cramping.

In view of my age, I need to keep in mind that I should take in more fluids than I feel I need when I'm engaged in physical activity. With aging, the ability to sense thirst decreases. Consequently, it's a good idea for older people to try to remember to drink more than they think they require, especially when exercising. Just how much is an interesting question.

The sight of people routinely carrying water bottles during daily activities reflects the response to a flood of information in recent years about the need to drink lots of water daily. Until not long ago, conventional wisdom, repeated over and over again in articles on health, had it that we all should drink at least eight glasses of water a day. Whenever I read that in the past, I thought it was nonsense. I'm gratified to know that relatively recent studies bear out my skepticism. Surveys of fluid intake by healthy adults have concluded that such a large amount is not necessary. They also have shown that the admonition that other beverages, caffeinated drinks in particular, should not be counted as part of the eight-glass total is also incorrect. New and more sensible guidelines do not provide a set amount of liquids to be consumed daily. Instead they state that most people get enough fluids by using their thirst as a guide. But again, to guard against dehydration the elderly should make a point of drinking more than their thirst dictates. Not a lot more necessarily, but somewhat more.

From the journal:

Day 24: Friday, May 31. Had breakfast before I left at 7:05, so there was no need to stop for a good while. The plan was for an easy ride on US 36 to Decatur, only 38 miles away, according to the map. The short ride would provide a test for my legs, and if they proved to be in good shape, I could ride farther. What I did not foresee was an unrelenting west wind that would slow me down to a crawl and, combined with the heat and high humidity, make the day less than enjoyable. The wind increased in intensity, and I was slowed con-siderably, once to five mph—and this was on a level road. By about noon I had stopped to rest three times, had gone only about 33 miles, and, with no place to get food or drink, was almost out of water and Gatorade. Finally I reached a convenience store and bought some water. Two miles later I reached a McDonald's on the outskirts of Decatur. Refueled with a hamburger, chocolate sundae, and water, water, water.

The streets of Decatur, a sizeable town (pop. 82,000, according to a sign I saw), were not bicycle friendly, but I navigated through them ok and headed for the motels that signs indicated were located on the western side of the city. Actually, they were several miles away. At 44 miles I found a Holiday Inn. The two young ladies at the reception desk inquired about my journey and were so impressed that they gave me a bottle of water. Then, after I had to get another key because the one they had given me didn't work, they sent two more bottles of water to my room (I must have looked pretty wiped out) and a plate of fruit. Maximum temperature today was 91°. Not an easy day, but, like each day's ride, it had good moments.

44 miles = 1,214 total

The need to drink a sufficient amount of liquids is especially necessary when the heat index—the combination of air temperature and relative humidity—is high. When that occurs, exertion can cause the blood temperature to rise above 98.6°. The heart rate goes up as the body tries to lose the extra heat by pumping more blood to enable capillaries in the upper layers of the skin to fill and draw heat off into the cooler air (unless the air temperature is greater than 98.6°). At the same time, water moves from the blood through the skin—sweating—which cools the body as the sweat evaporates, though not effectively when humidity is high. A high heat index will interfere with heat loss, resulting in overheating, which can cause discomfort at the very least and death at the very worst.

As people grow older, particularly as they reach their seventies and higher, they don't tolerate heat or respond to its dangers as well as when they were younger. Old people are more prone to suffer from heat exhaustion, heat stroke, or other forms of heat stress than younger people are. One reason for this is that aging reduces the body's ability to regulate its internal temperature when the heat index is high. In addition, because sweat glands don't function as efficiently as they do in younger people, there is less perspiration to help cool the body. Moreover, older people are more likely to have a chronic medical condition, like heart disease, that interferes with the body's responses to heat. And older people are more likely than younger to be taking medications that can impair the body's ability to regulate temperature or that can inhibit perspiration.

Even if in good health, the elderly need to be aware that, with aging, the body does not adjust as quickly or as well to temperature extremes. A hot muggy day should not mean an avoidance of exercise. However, everyone, especially the elderly, should take sensible precautions, such as restricting outdoor workouts to the coolest hours of the day, increasing the intake of water or sports drinks, and maintaining a slower-than-usual pace.

The beginning of summer was three weeks away, but already I was running into hot weather. Necessarily I rode much, sometimes most, of each day, but by not pushing my pace and taking in more liquid (although on occasion not enough to forestall leg cramps) I managed to avert heat exhaustion.

From the journal:

Day 25: Saturday, June 1. 7:05 departure after breakfast. Today's ride began well. Sky was overcast, temperature 72°, no wind. I followed US Rte 36, which within a mile merged with I-72. There I was, illegally on an interstate with no idea where else to go. With a sigh of relief, after eight miles I came to an exit, and found my way to the "Old US Rte 36", which runs east-west, paralleling I-72. A thunderstorm was developing to the northwest, but my route took me away from it. Made good time to Springfield, over 30 miles away. Just short of coming to the city, Rte 36 again merged with an interstate highway, this time I-55, and further along with I-72. As soon as I could, I got off the highway and picked my way through the downtown. After passing by the imposing state capitol, I rode for almost another hour before I got clear of the city. I followed directions to a road that after about a dozen miles took me back onto Old 36, which would take me to Jacksonville, my destination.

By the time I was clear of Springfield, I was riding into the face of a stiff westerly breeze. Soon the clouds broke, and before long it became hot and very humid. After riding for another hour and a half, I had covered over 50 miles since leaving Decatur. With my energy fading and figuring that making it to Jacksonville on my own would unduly exhaust me, I decided to hitchhike. After 15 minutes and no car yet in sight, I rode on for another mile, stopped, and waited again. This time, success! A young woman in a pickup truck stopped and took me to the center of Jacksonville [pop. 18,940], about ten miles down the road. I had lunch at a café then rode to the western edge of town, where I got a room at a motel—a little dingy, but not bad for $37—and called it a day at 2:30. Max. temperature today, 93°. Southeast winds forecast for tomorrow. Hope that's right.

55 miles (on the bike only—the ten miles by car don't count) = 1,269 total

Only twice on the journey did I feel compelled to try to hitch a ride, and only once, this day, did I succeed. Well, to be honest, there was one more time when I got a ride, in California; but I didn't actually hitchhike, and the ten-mile lift was back in the direction I came from, not in the direction I was headed.

The purist in me still feels guilty about not doing the entire distance using my own power, and I'm glad that my second attempt (in Kansas) failed. But in honesty, getting some help this day was not a bad idea. My journal does not wholly reflect how hot and tired I had become. Although I wrote that my energy was "fading," in reality I was bone tired and could well have been flirting with heat exhaustion. The temperature had climbed into the 90s, the air was very humid, I'd just about run out of water, and the headwind was gusting to over 20 miles an hour. Given all that, no doubt it was the better part of wisdom to seek a ride.

I hitchhiked a lot when I was a boy, and when I was in the navy I hitched rides home to San Luis Obispo when my ship was in port in San Francisco. In those days hitchhiking was common in America. The sight of both men and women, right thumb raised, standing on or plodding along the shoulder of the road, was in some places an everyday occurrence. There was no stigma attached to thumbing for rides, as there was in the 1920s, when hitchhikers were considered hobos or tramps. But beginning in the 1970s, hitchhiking declined considerably throughout the country. One reason for this was the widespread perception that life on the road was dangerous—a perception that gained credibility after some lurid murders of drivers or hitchhikers received considerable play in the media. In part because of such growing fears, laws were passed that circumscribed hitchhiking. While state laws rarely make the practice illegal, rules prohibiting hitchhiking in certain places, such as on major highways, are common and some local governments have banned it outright. Although hitchhiking has rebounded somewhat in the past decade or so, prohibitions and a general disinclination of motorists to pick up people seeking a lift continue to account for today's scarcity of hitchhikers.

The young woman who picked me up was, as I noted, driving a pickup, which had plenty of room in the back for the bike. I was tempted to tell her that although I appreciated her kindness, she was running a risk in picking up a hitchhiking stranger, but decided against it—didn't want to look a gift horse in the mouth, so to speak. Instead we talked about my trip and her life as a student at Jacksonville's Illinois College. Later, thinking about it, I realized that she was taking a non-existent to minimal risk in picking me up, since it wasn't likely that a serial killer would be riding a bicycle out in the middle of nowhere. Besides, a bedraggled, over-70 guy probably looked, and was, about as dangerous to her as a vegetable pizza.

From the journal:

Day 26: Sunday, June 2. Lost my Illinois map, but during breakfast at a café across the road from the motel, a waitress gave me the directions I needed. At 6:50 I took US 36 (now clear of I-72) out of Jacksonville for about 15 miles to Winchester, where I got on Illinois

Rte 106, which would take me to Hannibal, Missouri, via some small towns. Yesterday there were many dips and rises on my route but none very steep. Today, several miles out of Jacksonville I encountered rolling hills, which included a few long, fairly steep climbs, the worst of which was over a ridge on the western side of the Illinois River, about eight miles after Winchester. Although the predicted tailwind never materialized, I wasn't afflicted by a headwind today, except for an hour or so in the late morning.

After 20 more miles I came to Pittsfield, a town of about 4,000. Luckily, as it turned out, I didn't follow the sign there for a road to Hannibal. Instead I looked for and found a restaurant, where at lunch another patron told me that the way I was headed would take me to I-72, on which I couldn't ride, and that US 54 heading west out of town would, after four miles, get me back to Illinois Rte 106.

On that road at about mile 55, after a town called Barry, the terrain became more or less level again. Although today was not as hot as yesterday, an 87° maximum temperature combined with high humidity began taking a toll, and by mile 60 I was getting tired. However, the next eight miles went by quickly and, as I approached the Mississippi, Rte 106 intersected I-72. At the ramp onto I-72, I glanced at a sign that, I thought, contained the usual prohibition against use of the interstate highway by pedestrians, bicycles, and other small vehicles. I kept going, looking for another way across the river. Went a mile and a half on a road that dead-ended, giving me no choice but to return to the intersection with I-72. Once there I read the sign again, this time more carefully, and saw that bicycles were exempted from the prohibition.

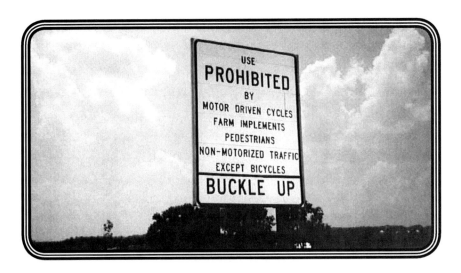

Sheepishly, after a few well-chosen words describing my stupidity, I crossed the bridge over the Mississippi and rode into Hannibal at 2:30. Got a room at a Best Western and went scouting around for a cold beer. Alas, it was Sunday, and in this part of Missouri alcoholic beverages were not to be had on the Sabbath. No mind, I was well satisfied to have reached and crossed the mighty Mississippi.

75 miles = 1,344 total

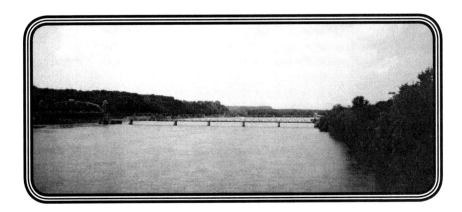

Crossing the Mississippi

In the preface of a book I wrote about Sudan, I said that because of their beauty and their place in human history, rivers have fascinated me. Because the Mississippi is a river so majestic and of such historical significance, riding over it was a special treat. I was glad on that Sunday to have time in Hannibal to wander around and take in some sights, including Mark Twain's boyhood home and the riverfront.

Road maps are produced with motorists in mind. Even the best road map can trip up a cyclist riding on a minor rural road. That happened to me this morning when my map did not show US 54 ruinning to the west of Pittsfield and intersectiing Rte 106. This was just one of the several times I rode extra miles because I took a wrong turn. A good rule of thumb is to ask locals for directions whenever there is even a scintilla of doubt about the route.

Back to the journal:

Day 27: Monday, June 3. It's 5:40 and I should be off in 15 minutes or so. Given that the forecast is for southwest winds at 10-15 mph, it's likely to be a long, hard day, and the earlier I start the better. Hope I find breakfast along the way before too long. Last night I had dinner with the first long-distance rider I have met on this trip. He was riding from Waynesville, Ohio, to Denver to see one of his sons.

5:15 pm. My worst enemy couldn't have planned a worse day. Well, I exaggerate, but not long after a good beginning, bad things started to happen. Left at 6 o'clock on the dot after coffee and a Gatorade Bar in my room. The one-mile hill up to US 36 wasn't too bad, and I felt in good shape. The next few miles included two more long hills, steep enough to require the granny gear, but the seven-foot paved shoulder was superb. Unfortunately, It lasted only five miles, after which the shoulder consisted of deep soft sand and gravel, totally unsuitable for riding. To make matters worse, US 36 was now two lanes with a fair amount of traffic, including many large trucks. I rode in the roadway when I could but frequently had to get over into the sand/gravel, risking a spill. At nine miles I stopped for breakfast at a truck stop, where a truck driver told me that beginning just down the road and continuing for 15 miles the shoulder would be ok. However, after that there would be no shoulder to speak of for quite a way. He was right. After the 15 miles, Rte 36 was without a shoulder again, a condition that, along with strong headwinds and some fairly difficult climbs, I had to put up with for several hours.

I have to admit that the ride was a bit dangerous at times because the wind force generated by passing trucks from both directions pushed me into the sand/gravel again now and then. A few times trucks came awfully close, and once the driver blasted his horn just as he whipped by me. What an s.o.b.

I relieved the stress by stopping for lunch about noon at Shelbina, a couple of miles south of US 36. Found a bar and grill and had a hamburger and a beer. Bought water and bananas at a supermarket,

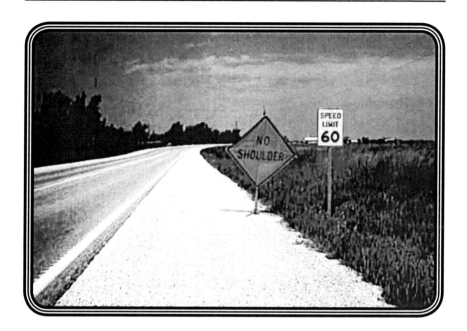

No kidding!

then went back to the grind. Began to tire when the wind increased during the afternoon, gusting to 28 mph. At around 3 o'clock, after I'd used up all my water and Gatorade, I reached the small town of Macon (pop. 5,500). The first exit from 36 brought me to fast-food places and a couple of motels. At a Hardee's, where my life was saved by a milkshake and lots of cold water, I learned that a motel with an adjoining restaurant was two miles farther west on 36. Arrived there just before 4. High temperature today was 88°. My calf muscles are cramping a bit.

67 miles = 1,411 total

In my journal, I didn't say much about the cyclist I met in Hannibal who was staying overnight in the same motel as I was. Bo Bradley was about 55, I'd say, well over six feet tall and weighing in the neighborhood of 230 pounds, he was a good-natured man who told me that a couple of years earlier, he tipped the scale at over 300. To lose weight, he took up exercising and discovered that he loved riding a bicycle. In the process of shedding excess pounds, he began riding progressively longer distances. On his current trip, from his home in Waynesville, Ohio, he had ridden to Kentucky to visit a son and now was heading for Denver to see another. Because of his size, he had a large, wide bike saddle of the kind I'm told is disdained by serious cyclists but is featured on rental cycles in tourist towns and enjoyed by older folks and others who like to pedal short distances. It worked fine for Bo. It would have been fun to ride with him, but we were headed in different directions.

Speaking of bicycle saddles, I had been attributing the almost constant discomfort and occasional outright pain in my backside to riding long miles on a saddle that just wasn't quite right for me. However, two days out of Hannibal, I discovered that the main, perhaps only, reason for the problem was a small boil. Ouch.

The nasty truck driver was an exception to the usually friendly, courteous truckers I encountered on the road. True, there were many times when their rigs came uncomfortably close as they passed me, but this tended to happen on narrow roads with ungenerous shoulders, posing situations in which the drivers could not ease to the left to give me more room. When this occurred, though, there probably was little if any danger, because the truck drivers knew what they were doing. Time and again, when they could they went out of their way to move leftward, putting a lot of space between their truck and me.

Car drivers, not truckers, were usually the villains of the disagreeable episodes that now and then briefly marred the journey. These incidents included derisory shouting, horn honking, angry looks, one-fingered salutes, and once a partly full soda can thrown at me. The weirdest happening took place in New Hampshire one afternoon when I was training. As I was riding along the coast on NH Rte 1-A, a car containing several young men passed me; they hollered and one gave me the finger. No big deal. They must have turned off the road and circled around, because a few minutes later they passed me again, going slowly. As they did, one of the guys stuck his bare behind out of the right-side rear window—I had been mooned! What they were trying to prove remains a mystery to me.

The unpleasant incidents during the trip were few and far between and only momentarily upsetting. It happened that Missouri was the state in which discourteous treatment was most prevalent. On the other end of the scale, drivers in western Kansas were the nicest I encountered anywhere.

From the journal:

Day 28: Tuesday, June 4. Got going at 6:50 following breakfast, continuing to head west on US 36. The first hour went well. The southwest wind was light, hills weren't too bad, and I made ten miles.

Then the wind freshened and the hourly mileage dropped. After three hours I'd gone only a total of 26 miles, and the going was getting even tougher. It was hilly and windy all day, putting a strain on my still somewhat rubbery legs. Had a burger and milkshake at Brookfield, 32 miles out. For the next few hours I plodded on, stopping to rest now and then. The sky was overcast, keeping the temperature down. Five miles from Chillicothe [pop. 8,968] it began to rain, hard at times. Just beyond the first off-ramp to the town I found a motel, the Grand River Inn, at 2:45. The wind had again made what would have been a relatively easy ride into another hard day. But no big problem, and I got in a fairly good total of miles today.

59 miles = 1,470 total

Towns or cities that have a claim to fame like to let the world know about it. A sign I read as I rode into Leroy, New York, proclaimed that Jell-O originated there, and one I saw as I entered Chillicothe touted that this was where sliced bread was invented (in 1928). Many places in the US—I don't know, maybe most— have something they brag about. When I was a boy in Pismo Beach, California, the town boasted that it was the home of the Pismo Clam. Many times I have driven through Castroville, California, "The Artichoke Capital of the World," and nearby Gilroy, "The Garlic Capital of the World." Over on the coast is Half Moon Bay, "The Pumpkin Capital of the World." My travels have taken me to Savannah, Georgia, "The Turf Grass Capital of the World;" Freeport, Illinois, "Pretzel City, USA;" Geneva, New

York, "Lake Trout Capital of the World;" Lompoc, California, "Flower Seed Capital of the World;" and Riverside, California, "Home of the World's Largest Paper Cup." I'm sure that I've passed through other places whose bragging rights I can't recall off the top of my head.

From the journal:

Day 29: Wednesday, June 5. According to the Weather Channel, it is now, at 6 am, 62° and the high today will only reach 75°. Although the sky is overcast, no rain is predicted. But, and this is the most pleasant prospect for me, winds will be light and from the northwest, not directly in my face.

To supplement the hotel's continental breakfast, I bought two Gatorade bars and some Gatorade at a convenience store. Got going at 7:05. Despite the light wind, because of hills, which appeared with regularity all day, I could average only about nine to ten mph most of the time. But that was better than yesterday with its incessant wind. When I got to Cameron, 38 miles from Chillicothe, I decided that my legs were now stronger and that I could make it to St. Joseph. After a burger and fries, I continued west on US 36. Some of the climbs over hills were a mile or longer but not steep. After I had gone 60 miles, the hills became infrequent and there were long stretches of level road. Approaching St. Joseph, I got into heavy traffic on what appeared to be a beltway. Saw the turnoff for Missouri 229, which I had been told would take me to a Holiday Inn. Riding up the on-ramp, after I passed through some dirt and road debris, the bike's front wheel suddenly went wobbly, and I realized I had a flat tire. Propped the bike up against the guardrail, took the wheel off and fixed the flat, no small feat, considering it was the first time I'd ever done it. Then I proceeded to the first off-ramp, which took me straight to the Holiday Inn. Will stay here tomorrow to take the bike to a bike shop to get my brakes fixed and to see a dermatologist, if I can get an appointment.

75 miles = 1,545 total

When in my journal I said I "fixed the flat," what I meant was that I replaced the tube. That night I did fix the flat by using a tube-repair kit. I located the hole in the damaged tube, abraded the area around it, and covered it with a patch. It held, and I was able to use the tube again.

Except for the ride from Richmond to Indianapolis on US Rte 40, for the most part I had been riding on US 36 for twelve days, beginning at Delaware, Ohio, and ending this day at St. Joseph. The approximately 650 miles I was on 36 was by far the longest distance I rode on any one highway. There were times, most notably in Missouri, when the road conditions were poor for bicycling. But for most of its length the highway gave me no heartburn, and riding on it was pleasant and safe. I have read that in the years since my journey, US 36 has been upgraded in Missouri and now is a four-lane divided highway throughout its course in the state.

From the journal:

Day 30: Thursday, June 6. Rode four miles to a bike shop, where I got new brake pads put on the rear wheel. In the afternoon a dermatologist looked at my legs and said the several red and purple splotches were not caused by sun exposure but instead were results of physical trauma. I guess I have been banging my shins with the bike's pedals. The visit to the doctor, along with getting a haircut, buying some sunscreen and an Allen wrench, and patching the punctured tire tube was pretty much my day in St. Joseph. Want to leave as early as I can tomorrow. I'll be headed southwest, and the forecast is for southerly winds becoming 25-30 mph in the afternoon.

After the dermatologist had pronounced that the marks on my legs were nothing to worry about if I kept them clean, he punctured the boil, to my great relief. Following my stops to get some sunscreen and an Allen wrench to replace one I had lost, I passed up a chance to stop at the house where, in 1882, Jesse James, living under the assumed name of Tom Howard, was killed by fellow bank robber Bob Ford—the "dirty little coward who shot Mr. Howard, and laid poor Jesse in his grave." Local tourism bills St. Joe as the place "Where the Pony Express started and Jesse James ended."

CHAPTER 7

Beautiful Kansas and the Great Plains

Kansas is a state of the Union, but it is also a state of mind, a neurotic condition, a psychological phase, a symptom, indeed, something undreamed of in your philosophy, an inferiority complex against the tricks and manners of plutocracy—social, political and economic.

William Allen White

Holcomb stands on the high wheat plains of western Kansas, a lonesome area that other Kansans call "out there."

Truman Capote

I don't know if I want to go to New York. They'll have to pay me a lot more money because I like it here in Kansas City.

Roger Maris

I know Kansas is a part of the Midwest, but because what I experienced there was, to my way of thinking, a marked change from the other Midwestern states, I'm devoting a separate chapter to Kansas in this narrative.

I had been riding for a month now. Most working Americans get only two weeks of vacation a year. This lack of enough free time for a cross-country bicycle trek closes the door to many or most working-age people who might want to give it a shot. And so for them, although physically it would be far better to set out before older age brings on diminished capacity, retirement is a pre-ride necessity.

Government-ordained and assisted retirement systems are relatively new. German Chancellor Otto von Bismarck, who set the retirement age at 70, introduced the first in the 1880s. Some years later the German government lowered the age to 65, the figure that was adopted by the Franklin D. Roosevelt administration when it brought in social security in 1935. Today, some 80 years later, aging and retirement in America remain strongly linked, and just as the elderly have to adjust to the physical changes that come with aging, those who leave the workforce have to adapt to a different set of circumstances.

While many new retirees feel liberated and ready to enjoy their new status, many others do not. Some of these are people whose sense of self-worth was centered on what they did for a living and who feel themselves diminished when their working life is over. Others simply love their work and don't want to quit. Increasingly in this day and age, a lot of people cannot financially afford to stop working (many baby boomers cite this as their reason for not retiring). Whatever causes their sense of loss, those who are forced into retirement need to recognize and resist reactions of distress or anger and, if they have a decent retirement income, look to the advantages of being out of the workforce.

Because I was about to reach the mandatory retirement age of 65, in the summer of 1995 I had to leave the Foreign Service. Between 1978 and 1995, I had been an ambassador three times and had held a relatively high-level position in the State Department. I believed I had reached a point in my career when my skills in diplomacy and management had grown to a level that made me more effective than ever, and I was angry at being forced to retire when I didn't want to. However, as the months went by the anger faded and I adjusted to a less strenuous, much less structured, and quieter existence.

I began to enjoy my freedom. I had time to write, and published two books. Julie and I did some traveling, and I did some pro-bono work regarding Sudan, which led to a part-time paid consultancy. In 1998-99, at the State Department's request, I spent the better part of a year heading the American embassy in Liberia. Two years later I had the time to prepare for and embark on my bicycle journeys. In 2005, a year after I had completed them, I accepted an appointment to head an international commission charged with defining and demarcating the boundaries of Abyei, a territory in dispute between Sudan and the about-to-become independent country of South Sudan. In 2009 I spent a couple of months in charge of our embassy in Zimbabwe. And beginning in 2007 I voluntarily restricted my freedom of action by becoming an elected member of the New Hampshire House of Representatives for two terms. All this is by way of illustrating that an active life for me did not end with retirement.

From the journal:

Day 31: Friday, June 7. The last leg of the ride through Missouri on US 36 yesterday had been on a very good roadway, a four-lane divided highway with a smooth-surfaced four-foot wide shoulder. US Rte 59 out of St. Joe was just as good, at least initially. I left the Holiday Inn at 6, not long before the sun came up. Rode out on 6th Street, which became US 59 and took me clear of the city after five miles. From there until I reached the Missouri River, at mile 24, the land was gloriously flat, a harbinger, I hoped, of Kansas. Did the 24 miles in two hours and stopped in Atchison, Kansas for breakfast after crossing the river.

Soon afterward the road was under construction, and for 28 miles I rode on newly laid asphalt, which was as smooth as silk. No shoulder but very little traffic. Only problem was that this part of Kansas is not flat. The hills weren't steep, but I was riding into a headwind that, as predicted, increased in strength steadily throughout the morning. US 59 turned south, and I continued southwest on Kansas Rte 4.

The wind and the hills slowed my progress considerably, but by noon I'd covered 50 miles. Although there was a bed and breakfast at Valley Falls, I decided to press on to Topeka. Had a hamburger and milkshake at a small restaurant at Meriden. No milkshakes on the menu, but the lady who waited on me said she'd make one, and was it ever delicious. The traffic increased as I got closer to Topeka, and I was often buffeted by the blast of air from oncoming trucks. One truck knocked a pebble into the air that hit me on the arm with enough force to break the skin. Glad it didn't hit me in the face.

At 70 miles from St. Joseph, I turned west on US 24, finally turning away from the headwind, and quickly covered four miles to Kansas Avenue, which took me into downtown Topeka. Checked into a Ramada Inn at about 4. Sky was clear all day, maximum temperature 86°.

On this trip I've found that the quality of chain or franchise hotels and motels has varied from place to place. This Ramada Inn, for example, has seen better days and compares unfavorably to the two other Ramada Inns where I've stayed, both excellent. I don't know if the state of this one had anything to do with the fact that it was all but deserted when I went to the bar for a beer and then later at dinner, for the occupancy of almost all the places I've stayed in so far has been pretty low, no matter what their appearance. Guess it's because my route is mostly far off the beaten path for tourists.

80 miles = 1,625 total

The ride from St. Joseph to Topeka was the kind of day any cyclist would enjoy, not completely easy, but not particularly difficult. It included 28 miles of unalloyed pleasure produced by the supersmooth surface of a relatively flat highway, a thirst quenching ultra-delicious milkshake, and a new city to see.

This was also a day of examples of the good nature of people I met on the road. Perhaps it was pity or admiration that prompted the lady at Meriden to go to the trouble to make me a milkshake, but I think it was just plain niceness. In Topeka, it was early, about six, when I went to dinner in the hotel restaurant. I was the only person seated. Perhaps I looked a bit lonely in the large dining room, and the waitress, a woman of about 50, made every effort to make me feel welcome. She advised me which of the menu entrees were best, gave me information about Topeka, and exchanged life histories with me. We talked about our respective families. I remarked on how tough a job waitressing must be, but she said she liked her job, especially because she met interesting people. It didn't pay much, but her husband worked and, she said, "We get along just fine." A gracious, considerate lady and a delight to talk with.

From the journal:

Day 32: Saturday, June 8. I won't call this a pleasant day, but it was not without interest. [My friend Bruce McCurdy had an art professor in college who often, upon regarding a student's work, would comment elliptically, "It is not without interest."] I left the hotel at 5:50, and a half-hour and six miles later stopped at a Denny's for breakfast. Back on the road at 7, I kept going south on US-75, headed for the junction with US 50, where I planned to turn west to Emporia. The prediction for strong southerly winds proved, unfortunately for me, only too correct, and I was feeling a bit weary after five hours. When, at mile 45, I reached the junction, I found that US 50 merged with I-35 and that bicyclists are prohibited on I-35. What to do? I decided I had no choice but to hitchhike, which I set out to do at the on-ramp to I-35, but after a fruitless hour gave up. In a down mood, I went to a truck stop on the other side of the interstate, where I got a sandwich, lots of liquid, and some more rest, adding to that which I'd accrued while hitchhiking. I learned that "Old Rte 50" was two miles south and paralleled I-35. Revived, and with my equanimity restored, I pedaled there and turned west. What a difference it was not to have to battle the headwind. Reached Emporia in a little more than two hours. Stopped for water and directions at a convenience store and continued west through the city until I came to a good motel. Arrived at 5:30—a long day but a good one. I'm glad the hitchhiking didn't pan out. Had I succeeded, I would have regretted not making it to Emporia all on my own. And since I could not count any miles I didn't accumulate under my own power, the day's total would have been only 45.

78 miles = 1,703 total

Day 33: Sunday, June 9. Breakfast at the motel, on the road at 6:50. Bought some Powerade at a gas station. Had a bottle of it yesterday and found its bouquet of Kiwi irresistible. The forecast was for a continued strong southerly wind with gusts up to 30 mph. Riding west on US 50 out of Emporia, I covered 12 miles the first hour, but hills slowed me down somewhat the second. At about mile 25, a half hour past Strong City, US 50 bent to the southwest, and once more I found myself struggling with the wind. Consequently, I looked forward to reaching, a few miles down the road, a junction with Kansas Rte 150, which ran due west and would get me out of the headwind. But at the junction a sign said that 150 was closed, which meant that to get to Marion, on the way to McPherson, my intended

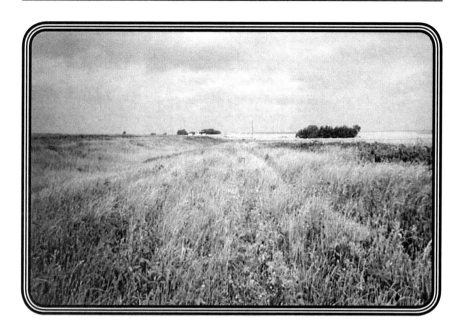

Detour

objective for the day, I would have to continue going southwest on Rte 50 for 17 miles and then take US 77 north back to Kansas 150. Not only would this mean adding nine or ten miles to the ride, but also I would be going 17 miles into the teeth of the now fiercely blowing wind. Mulling this over, I concluded that although 150 was closed to cars, most likely a bike could get through, so I decided to take my chances on 150.

The first obstacle was an impassable excavation for a bridge. Pushed the bike off the road into a field of waist-high grass and, with a herd of cows looking on, walked with it for a few minutes until I found a way across a muddy ditch back to the road. Soon discovered that it would not be a matter of just a few excavations, but that the entire road was torn up and being reconstructed. At times I had to

push the bike over rubble, but generally I could ride slowly over a
rough clay-gravel surface. In two hours I went about eight miles,
after which the road improved and I made better time, reaching the
beginning of a recently laid concrete roadway that extended the rest
of the way to the intersection with US 77, where Kansas 150 became
US 56. Five miles farther on, I came to Marion, where I stopped for
a sandwich and Coke before pressing on at a pretty good clip for 37
miles to the western outskirts of McPherson [pop, 13,770], which I
reached at 4 pm. Found a motel with a restaurant next door. To my
dismay, I learned that here, as in Hannibal, Sunday blue laws meant
there would be no cold beer for the weary traveler.

81 miles = 1,784 total

Currently, the prevailing opinion is that plain water is an adequate rehydration beverage if exercise lasts less than an hour and perspiration is not excessive. However, using only water is not recommended for longer-term strenuous activities, and I supplemented bottles of water with either Gatorade or Powerade.

Gatorade, developed at the University of Florida in 1965, was the first of the sports drinks designed to replenish electrolytes lost through sweat during heavy exercise. The hot and humid days of Florida summers hatched a realization that there was a need for something more than just water and salt tablets. It took a while for sports drinks to catch on, but beginning in 1991 consumption of Gatorade, and soon after Powerade and other sports drinks, took off. They now are universally accepted as enhancers of prolonged exertion, especially when the heat index is high. Most sports drinks meet the standard of consisting of four to six percent of carbohydrate and at least 80-110 milligrams of sodium per eight-ounce serving. So the choice of which drink to use can be made on the basis of which one tastes best.

The acceptance of drinking liquids during exercise was a quantum leap from an earlier belief that athletes needed to abstain from drinking water during practice to avoid bloating and to make them mentally tougher. Other myths that prevailed included the view that weight training would make athletes muscle-bound and slow and that football players would be aided by eating steak and potatoes before games.

I well remember that in the late 1940s, when I played high school junior-varsity football, and the 1950s, when I was on the football team at UC Santa Barbara, the standard operating procedure disallowed water during practice. On very hot days we were permitted to take a swig of water and swish it around in our mouth but not to swallow it.

Shrimp that I was, weight training in college would definitely have been to my advantage, but coaches and ball players didn't even consider it. As for a steak dinner before a game, it probably didn't help but most likely did no harm. And a free steak dinner at restaurant was a most welcome windfall.

Kansas has no state control over the sale of alcoholic beverages, but McPherson remains one of the state's communities that prohibit sales on Sundays. Beginning in 1617 in Connecticut, for more than 300 years blue-law restrictions on Sunday activities were common in America. Based on Christian religious beliefs, blue laws were designed to counter behavior that was regarded as immoral. In the early days of their existence, some blue laws meted out draconian punishments to sinners, including whipping and even death for violating the Sabbath.

By the 20th century the excessive puritanical punishments of blue laws had been abolished, but Sabbath restrictions of one kind or another remained in many states. Older Americans can remember when, by law, virtually all stores and businesses were closed on Sundays. Statewide restrictions on certain activities on Sundays are fairly rapidly being eliminated but still are on the books of more than a dozen states. Activities that are most singled out for restrictions are alcoholic beverage sales and, curiously, car sales and hunting. In states that have eliminated bans on Sunday booze sales there have been two discernible effects: an increase in state revenues and a decrease in church attendance and donations.

From the journal:

Day 34: Monday, June 10. 6 am. The Weather Channel says we now have 75°, 87 percent humidity, and a south wind of 18 mph. Prediction is for 95-100 degrees, continued high humidity, stronger wind.

Got on the road at 6:50 and reached Lyons, 33 miles west of McPherson, three hours later. Had breakfast at a McDonald's, no other option being available. Thought the next 30-odd miles to Great Bend wouldn't be much of a strain. But the wind, even though it was from my left side instead of dead ahead, miles of slightly upward inclines, and increasing heat hindered my progress. Except for a short spell when the road had a seven-foot shoulder, US 56 between McPherson and Great Bend offered only a one- to two-foot shoulder. That was better than a lot of the roads I've ridden over, but this two-lane highway has a lot of truck traffic, and the blasts of wind generated by fast-moving large trucks knocked me about from time to time. It was 98° when I pulled into Great Bend [pop. 15,345]. Once in town, I had the front brakes adjusted at a bicycle shop and bought battery-operated flashing red lights for the back of the bike.

65 miles = 1,849 total

After I crossed the Missouri the land began gradually and steadily to slope upward after over 1,300 miles of no appreciable overall change in altitude. Atchison's elevation is 950 feet, Topeka's 1,000, and Emporia's 1,150. My next day's ride from there took me to McPherson, which sits at 1,504 feet. The elevation of Tribune, my last stop in Kansas, is 3,616 feet. This upslope would continue to about 6,000 feet as I rode through eastern Colorado on into the foothills of the Rocky Mountains.

In the vicinity of McPherson, I entered America's Great Plains, which sweep south from well inside the Canadian interior across parts of ten American states, extending from Montana to the Texas-Mexico border. When the last great continental glacier was spread to its maximum extent, spruce forest had appeared as far south as Kansas and deciduous forest covered the land farther south. When the ice retreated to the north, the trees went with them, and ever since the Great Plains has been a treeless grassland.

The Rocky Mountains mark the Plains' western boundary. The eastern boundary is arbitrarily and variously demarcated by the 1,500-foot contour line, or the 98th or 100th meridians of longitude, or, the most amorphous, a line (isohyet) marking the approximate western limit of rainfall of 20 or more inches. Riding into the Great Plains on a bicycle and therefore seeing the landscape's changes unfold literally foot by foot, I could agree with the assertion that in Kansas the beginning of the Great Plains becomes apparent along a line running north-south just west of Salina or, where I was riding 30 miles farther south, near McPherson. From Emporia almost to Strong City I had ridden through the rounded, gently rolling Flint Hills. They gave way to more level surfaces, and after leaving McPherson I came to a broad flat plateau that stretched out ahead as far as I could see. I was now in a part of the vast area that was home to countless thousands of bison before their virtual extermination by white hunters in the 1870s and to the nomadic, horse-riding Plains Indian tribes before white men drove them out.

It was possible, if I made an effort to blot out the highway and other signs of human activity, to imagine how unplowed grasslands, filled with grazing bison, might have looked before their wholesale slaughter took place. However, because the land today differs so much from what it was in the nineteenth century, imagination has to work very hard to visualize how the Great Plains appeared to the white settlers coming to them in the 1830s and for some years afterwards. Although forests had given way to croplands for over 200 years, much of the eastern United States was still forested, heavily in places, and trees were a common feature of farms and towns. To travelers and settlers from the east the contrast between it and the treeless, trackless plains was stark, and to many frightening.[10]

From the journal:

Day 35: Tuesday, June 11. Leg cramps again last night, this time in the muscle along the left side of the left leg's shinbone. That and the need to give the chafing on my behind, probably a result of yesterday's heat, a chance to heal, add up to a need to rest here in Great Bend today. For a variety of reasons, including the amazingly bad food in its restaurant, I don't like the large-chain motel where I'm staying and will move across the street to another.

Went to the post office to mail my radio and headphones home. Used them briefly only once in Indiana and once in Kansas. The radio worked well in both instances and listening to it didn't prevent me from hearing approaching traffic. Yet it's clear that I won't use it enough to justify carrying it any longer.

10　S.C. Gwynne, *Empire of the Summer Moon* (New York, Scribner, 2010) 38-39.

As it turned out, it was a good idea to give my legs a rest. Once more, overexertion and dehydration were logical causes. But you don't have to ride a bike for the better part of a day to experience leg cramps at night. Aging is definitely a factor, for studies show that about 70 percent of adults older than 50 are at times afflicted with nocturnal leg cramps. This can happen even to healthy individuals who have exercised for years. As for me, dehydration was undoubtedly the culprit, for in view of the amount of energy I was putting into my daily rides and the hot weather I was encountering, I should have been drinking more each day I was riding.

A word on motels: As I noted in the journal entry for the day that ended in Topeka, motel chains do not necessarily mean uniformity of quality, and the disparities I encountered, for instance the one this day in Great Bend, bore that out. On this and later bicycle trips I often stayed at non-chain, mom-and-pop motels. As a rule less expensive than the chains, they ranged from excellent to barely tolerable. Still, my needs were minimal—a clean bed and a shower the only real requirements. So I really didn't mind the less-than-best quality and I loved some of the bargain rates, which in one town was only $21.

From the journal:

Day 36: Wednesday, June 12. Oreo cookies and coffee for ignition. Underway at 6, with the bike's new red backlights blinking on and off until the sun dispelled the semi-darkness and I turned them off. A couple of miles outside of town, US Rte 56 turned southwest and I continued west on Kansas Rte 96. The predicted westerly winds never materialized. Instead there was no wind at all. It was a beautiful day. A bright blue sky was partly obscured by towering cumulus clouds. To the west thunderstorms were unleashing chain lightning that flashed down to the earth.

Clouds kept the temperature down most of the morning, and even after they dissipated, the day wasn't that hot (max. temp. 80°). Along the way there were a fair number of gradual upward inclines and a couple of steep ones that forced me to use the granny gear, but the ride today was mostly over flat ground and I made reasonably good time.

Thirty-two miles from Great Bend, I stopped for breakfast at Rush Center (pop. 207), pleased to find a small café there. The two other patrons in the café were cyclists, a father and son, Bill and Andy Merritt from Glastonbury, Connecticut, who are riding from Yorktown, Virginia, headed for Oregon, then down to San Francisco. A bicycle tours company, Adventure Cycles, has a west-east tour, the TransAmerica Trail, which they are following in reverse—as I am, but only from Rush Center to Pueblo, Colorado. At Pueblo they will go north and I'll go northwest. I didn't ask to ride with them since, pretty sure that they would be making better time than I could, I didn't want to hold them back. They left while I was finishing breakfast.

By noon I had gone 61 miles and shortly afterward I was in Ness City [pop. 1,534]. Rode through town, found the post office, mailed some postcards, and was told that the Derrick Inn is the only hotel in town. Ended the day's ride at 1 pm. Kansas Rte 96 has proven to be a fine two-lane road with an excellent two-foot shoulder. Some trucks, but traffic is much lighter than it was on US 56.

66 miles = 1915 total

Many years before, on two different occasions I drove through Kansas on my way from California to Washington, DC. My recollection is that because I found the scenery blah, I wanted to get the Kansas leg of the trip behind me as soon as possible.

Crossing the state on a bicycle was an entirely different experience. For one thing, the flatness that had bored me was now most welcome. The towns themselves, though lacking in charm, had a certain character, reflecting the stark lines of the countryside. My abiding memory of the Kansas I rode through on my way west is the beauty of the yellow, brown, and springtime green of the earth vividly in contrast to the color of the sky, now deep blue, now filled with the roiling, swollen lower reaches of thunderclouds. One day in particular the combination of vast plains and a countryside of changing colors under a lowering sky was a sight to behold.

The grain silos and elevators that rose slowly from the horizon as I made my way through south central and southwestern Kansas and on into eastern Colorado provided a dramatic contrast to the flat countryside. From McPherson, Kansas, to Eads, Colorado, about 300 miles, I passed many of these massive structures. Appearing first as a faint break on the skyline, they took shape gradually as I pedaled toward them. The taller ones were as many as 15 miles from me when I first caught sight of their tops, and an hour or more would pass before I would reach them.

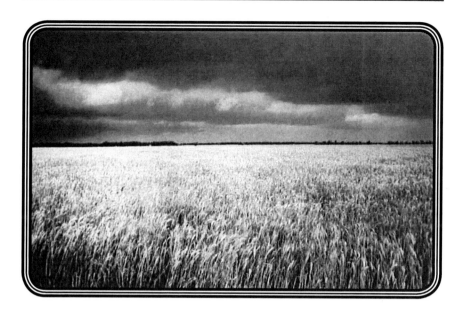

Between Great Bend and Ness City

Continuation of Wednesday's journal:

9 pm. My cell phone is out of whack and I won't be able to get it fixed until I get to Pueblo, 271 miles from Ness City. I could try to ride 79 miles to Leoti tomorrow and 80 to Eads the next day, Friday. From Eads it's a two-day ride to Pueblo, which means I would arrive there Sunday, when the Verizon store I need might well be closed. Alternatively, I could go 55 miles to Scott City tomorrow, about 50 to Tribune Friday, and 62 to Eads on Saturday, arriving in Pueblo Monday. I would prefer the first alternative, but I think two long rides in a row in the hot and humid weather might not be a good idea and have decided on the five-day alternative. I should get into Pueblo early Monday afternoon, when I can get my cell phone fixed and have some work done on the bike.

Day 37. Thursday, June 13. One of the thunderstorms in the area today dumped a lot of rain on Ness City shortly before I left town at 6 am. A mile down the road, I had to stop to readjust the saddle, which I had tinkered with last night. After eight miles, the rain began to fall. Lightning flashing directly ahead was worrisome. So was the onset of hail, but that lasted less than a minute and after four more miles I was clear of the rain. I had stopped to put my sweatshirt on under my windbreaker and now kept both of them on because, with a brisk NNE wind blowing and a drop in temperature, it was cold.

As near as I can tell from the map, the gain in altitude between Ness City and Scott City, 55 miles to the west and my destination today, is about 700 feet. The upward slope of the road was noticeable from time to time, but only a problem once when it coincided with a temporary headwind. Had breakfast at Dighton, 31 miles out of Ness City, at 9 and continued on to Scott City [pop. 3,855], still on KS Rte 96, arriving at noon. Scouted around town for a grocery store, motels, and places to eat before choosing the Airliner Motel ($34, tax included), which has an adjoining restaurant.

60 miles = 1975 total

Getting wet in a thunderstorm is no big deal. Being bombarded by small pellets of hail could be uncomfortable, however, and by golf-ball size hail dangerous. But lightning poses the greatest danger to a cyclist caught in a thunderstorm. Advice on what to do is easy to come by and easy to follow.

If you hear thunder, whether or not you see lightning, look for safe shelter immediately. If you are under or near tall trees, get away from them as fast as you can. If you find yourself on a hill with exposure to the sky, head downhill. Ride to a low spot away from trees, fences, and poles, but be sure that the lower area is not liable to be flooded in a heavy downpour. Look for shelter, such as a sturdy building, barn, store, or overpass. Don't believe that the rubber tires of a bike offer protection; they do not. And remember that lightning remains a danger even when a thunderstorm is dissipating or has passed by.

From the journal:

Day 38: Friday, June 14. This was a day when I could have ridden 100 miles, or at least I felt that I could, but instead I stuck to my plan to reach Pueblo on a Monday rather than a Sunday and I settled for fewer miles. The temperature was down to 52° when I left Scott City at 7:10, and I wore tights over my riding shorts and a long-sleeve T-shirt over a regular T-shirt, topped off with my windbreaker. A perfect day—cool air, no wind, and a clear blue sky with not even a wisp of a cloud. Kansas Rte 96 has become my favorite road so far, given its smooth surface, good shoulders, sparse traffic, and lack of any hills to speak of. The gradual rise in altitude continued to be a factor, but I made good progress this morning, reaching Tribune [pop. 835] in less than four hours. Some bike riders might find Kansas boring, but I don't. Its very flatness—the immensity of the plain, extending to the horizon ahead and to both right and left for hour after hour—impresses me deeply. Today the juxtaposed colors of blue sky, golden wheat, green corn stalks, and brown plowed fields were striking. And man, do I appreciate the absence of hills.

When I checked in at Tribune's lone motel, the Trail's End ($33.89, including tax), the lady at the desk said she'd have to clean a room for me because it was so early, only 10 am. I hadn't realized that Mountain Time begins about ten miles east of Tribune. Rode into town to visit a food store, the library, and a café.

50 miles = 2,025 total

It wasn't until after the Civil War that Kansas began to attract sizeable numbers of settlers. Most of today's Kansas towns were founded in the 1870s and 1880s as thousands of people—encouraged by promoters of one stripe or another and attracted by the prospect of free land under the terms of the 1862 Homestead Act—arrived to begin new lives. Many stayed, but thousands left, unable to make a living on a 160-acre homestead or defeated by drought or driven insane by loneliness and the incessant winds.

The peak of rural population in the Great Plains came not long after the towns were established. A period of some stability followed but did not last, as a seemingly inexorable decrease in the number of inhabitants ensued. Although the overall population of the Great Plains has increased since 1950, from the Dakotas to the Texas Panhandle the rural Great Plains has been losing people for 80 years, a gradual but thus far steady demographic decline.

I find it sad that Tribune, whose appearance I found appealing, may well be one of the dying towns on the Great Plains.

A comparison of 2000 and 2010 census data for the seven towns I passed through beginning with McPherson, Kansas, and ending with Ordway, Colorado, gives no rise to optimism. It shows that only Great Bend, the largest town, gained in population (by 4 percent). Of the two other larger towns, Scott City stayed even and McPherson went down by 4.5 percent. The four smaller towns all saw substantial population losses—Ness City 6 percent, Tribune 11 percent, Ordway 13 percent, and Eads 18 percent. Efforts by municipal and state government to revive towns like these have met with little if any success.

From the journal:

Day 39: Saturday, June 15. Last night as I was about to walk across the highway to the sandwich shop at the truck stop, the motel's owner, a fit-looking man about 45-years old, asked me if I'd like some chicken and corn that he was about to cook on an outdoor grill. Sure, I said, and an hour later he served me up two large pieces of chicken, an ear of corn, some tomatoes, onions, and mushrooms, and a bottle of beer. Best food I've had in many days. He's a cyclist himself, and after I had eaten we talked about how he came to this small town, his bicycle trips, and the politics of Greeley County, which is solidly Republican, having given George W. Bush 78 percent of its votes to Al Gore's 18 percent in the 2000 election. One thing I told him was that here in western Kansas I've been struck by how friendly motorists have been, many of them waving to me as they've driven by.

Now that I'm on the eastern edge of a new time zone, sunrise is earlier, 5:12 this morning. Had a ham, egg, and cheese sandwich and coffee for breakfast at the truck stop and got on the road at 6:10. For three hours there was a stiff wind coming in toward my left shoulder, and I had to work hard to average 9 mph. Sixteen miles west of Tribune I crossed into Colorado, and before long the quality of the road changed for the worse. The asphalt was heavily embedded with pebbly small-gauge gravel, raising, I thought, a danger of punctures. The gradual rise in altitude continued (Tribune's elevation is about 3,600 feet, Eads' about 4,200). There were some climbs, as the road crossed a succession of ridges running north to south. The temperature rose into the high 80s, and I needed all the water and Gatorade I was carrying. Just before Eads, the rough surface of Rte 96 (now Colorado Rte 96) gave way to a wonderfully smooth concrete roadway. Arrived at Eads at 12:15.

58 miles = 2,083 total

A frequent question I hear from people who ask me about the journey is how I coped with the solitude as I rode between towns. Sometimes on two-lane roads with narrow or no shoulders and a fair amount of traffic, of necessity I would be focused on keeping as far to the right as I could manage safely and not be thinking about anything else. There were times when my thoughts were centered on beautiful scenery, but there were also days when, for hours on end, the view was far from captivating. Having no pre-set strategy for dealing with instances like these, I let my mind wander to a theme or topic or idea, which I would pick up on and proceed to think about. For example, I relived—with as much detail as I could dredge up—aspects of my life, such as growing up in Pismo Beach and San Luis Obispo, my school days from grade school through university, my fours years in the navy, the courtship of Julie, our marriage, our children, and the many different places where we lived abroad and in the United States. I mined my memory for music, both words and melodies, which I would sing in my head, or aloud if I wasn't exerting myself battling a strong wind or steep hills. I would jot down sights or events to write in my journal at the end of the day, or something I wanted to identify, like a kind of sagebrush along the road or the name of a nearby mountain range.

I suppose it might have been restful to think of nothing at all as I rode along, but I don't have that ability.

CHAPTER 8

Colorado and the Rockies

I'm a grandmother with dogs and nice friends here in the Rocky Mountains. Ever see the movie A River Runs Through It? That's where I live. It's beautiful, no two ways about it.

Margot Kidder

The mountains are calling and I must go.

John Muir

From the journal, a continuation of day 39 entry:

The Country Manor Motel here in Eads is the third in a row having a room for less than $35, and does that ever appeal to my frugality. Big thunderstorm and heavy downpour late this afternoon. Forgot to mention that not long after I entered Colorado, there was a sudden and, to me, dramatic change in the vegetation, as cultivated farmland was replaced by sagebrush grazing land dotted in some places with cactus plants. It was as if a line between the Midwest and the West had fairly abruptly been crossed.

At the motel I met two men and two women, all four appearing to be in their thirties, who are following much of Adventure Cycle's TransAmerica Trail, but, like the Merritts, in the opposite direction, going from east to west instead of Adventure Cycle's west-east route. They won't hook north to Oregon from Pueblo, Colorado, as Bill and Andy, were intending to do. Alternatively, the four will leave the Adventure Cycle course at Pueblo, Colorado, and ride through Utah and Nevada en route to San Francisco. We had dinner together, and afterward I went over their maps and decided I couldn't follow their route, which includes some long (100 or more miles) stretches having no places at all for food or drink. For them that is not a problem, since they have a van and take turns driving it. Thus they carry little besides water on their bikes and can eat up more miles per day than I can. And they don't have to worry about not being able to reach a place to stay, for they can simply put the bikes on the van and drive to the next available lodging. So, for now at least, I'll stick to the route I have chosen.

Like Tribune, Kansas, the tiny town of Eads is a county seat of a thinly populated county. In 2000 Eads had almost half of Kiowa County's total population of 1,622. The number of its inhabitants in that year, 747, would decrease to 609 ten years later. The town's appearance may have given a clue as to why Eads seems moribund. Its non-descript buildings and general ambience had nothing that would attract newcomers or hold its residents, especially young people. Even in good economic times, good jobs in Eads would be at a premium.

One way to make a long-distance bike ride is to pay a fee to a commercial cycling-tours company. The cost will vary depending on the length of the tour, whether it is fully or only partly supported and whether at least some of the overnight stays are in campgrounds instead of motels or hotels. One that I checked out on the Internet before leaving New Hampshire offered full support, including luggage transportation, bike repairs, medical care if needed, accommodations booked at AAA-rated hotels and motels, breakfast and dinner, and mid-ride snacks. One advantage is that you use a road bike instead of a heavier touring bike, like mine, and carry little besides fluids for drinking. A result of this is longer distances ridden per day. Another is the certainty of lodging. A third is the companionship that riding with a group of people provides. However, the price tag—up to $8,500 for a cross-country tour in 2002 and no doubt higher now—is a bigger expense than a lot of riders would want to shoulder.

Another option is the one chosen by the four people I met in Eads. They had the advantage of knowing that they would be traveling with friends, with whom they no doubt knew they were compatible, something that is not a sure thing when riding on a commercial tour. A disadvantage, at least to my way of thinking, is that, because each of them drove the van at times, none could say they had ridden the whole distance across the country.

Although I looked at the material on websites of a few commercial tours, and expect it would be fun to ride on them, I never seriously considered signing on with one to make my cross-America ride. I wanted to do my own planning and make the ride on my own. To do otherwise would not have been nearly as challenging or, I believe, fulfilling.

From the journal:

Day 40: Sunday, June 16. Fortunately I had breakfast before I left Eads, since it turned out that the only town between Eads and my destination, Ordway, that had a place to eat was Sugar City, 57 miles away. That some of the tiny towns along Rte 96 in western Kansas and eastern Colorado are dying was evident in the many closed-down businesses, like cafés, I saw along the road as I passed by.

Almost the entire ride today was through country that appeared to be suitable only for grazing cattle. For more than four hours, a southwest wind slowed me down. The highway's surface was pebbly, as it was yesterday, but older and more compacted and seemed to me to be no threat to bicycle tires. From roughly mile 13 to mile 18 there was a steady, gradual increase in elevation. After I had ridden 45 miles, the wind began to shift, and soon I had a light tail wind, at last! Passed a cyclist going the other way. He had no load on his bike, so I assumed he was not going far. But a mile or so down the road, I came upon a young woman in an SUV who told me she was his wife and his "support team" on his cross-country trip. Armed with reading material and the car's radio, she seemed quite at ease with what I would have found utterly monotonous, but what for her, I guess, was truly a labor of love.

In Ordway I rode up to the Ordway Hotel, the only lodging in town. Signed in and paid $10 for a room on the second floor. No elevator, so I unloaded the bike and hauled it up the stairs. There was no bathroom in the room. I'd have to use one down the hall. But, what the heck, for $10.... After getting settled in the room I noticed that the bed had no pillow and, after a quick check, no sheets. The lady who runs the hotel explained that she figured I wanted the bare-bones accommodation preferred by cyclists, which probably meant that they were young and on a tight budget. She said that if I wanted, I could have a regular room, which included an attached bathroom. With alacrity, I chose the more expensive option. Had to pay an additional $11, total $21, an all-time low, or from the standpoint of satisfaction, high. The room was small and spartan but met all my needs. It even had a window a/c unit. Went out for lunch at a mom-and-pop café and chowed down on some delicious fried chicken. And now here I am in my room, showered, no longer starving, and happily watching the US Open golf tournament on TV. Will need to get underway early again tomorrow to continue to beat the worst of the heat. The high temperature in Pueblo tomorrow is slated to be 97° or higher.

63 miles = 2,146 total

Ordway looked neater, cleaner and generally more prosperous than Eads. Nevertheless, it too would see its population decrease, from 1,248 in 2000 to 1,080 in 2010.

For the past few days the maximum temperature had been in the mid-80s, but the forecast for next two days was for extreme heat, and I would have to be extra careful to drink plenty of liquids. To reduce the amount of time spent riding during the hottest time of the day, I needed to get on the road as early as possible. If I were to strictly follow medical advice for the elderly to forestall heat exhaustion or heat stroke, I would have to sharply reduce physical activities and even stay indoors for a good part of the day. I was hardly in a position to do either. Yet, as it happened, although severe heat did hasten the onset of weariness during a long ride, the high temperatures didn't unduly affect me, I assume because I was by now in pretty good physical condition.

From the Journal:

Day 41: Monday, June 17. It was cool, 52°, when the day began and very hot when it ended. My startup fuel was a banana. I was disappointed that nothing was open early in the morning in Ordway or in Crowley or Olney Springs, six and eleven miles down the road. Five miles farther on, an hour and a half after my 5:45 departure from Ordway, I turned south off Colorado Rte 96 and, crossing over the Arkansas River, rode two miles to Fowler to look for a place to eat. Unlike the other towns I've seen these past few days, Fowler had an attractive downtown—a mixture of late 19th and early 20th century western architecture along with more contemporary buildings, and a generally spruced-up appearance. Had a fine breakfast at the first café I spotted.

Between Ordway and Olney Springs I had had a moment of elation when I caught my first glimpse of the Rockies on the western horizon. A west wind began to blow at 9 am and of course slowed me down, but, I'm happy to say, the wind never reached the 10-20 mph velocity predicted by the Weather Channel.

Back on Rte 96, several miles east of Pueblo, for the first time since I left home a dog (a black Lab) left the confines of his yard and made a run at me. I'm not sure he was serious, but he made a pretty good show of wanting a piece of my right leg. My defense: "Bad dog, go home!" Whether intimidated by this display of ferocity or not, he shied off and went back to his yard. After I reached Pueblo (elevation 4,500 feet) at 11:45, the traffic on Rte 96 soon became so heavy that I took the first off-ramp I came to, which put me into a middle-class residential area, where I promptly got lost. Pueblo is a relatively big city (pop. about 102,000), and I had no idea where I was. Finally I came upon a Dairy Queen, where I had a delicious strawberry milk-shake and got directions to The Great Divide, the bicycle shop I was looking for. Once there, I replaced the saddle with a new one—there must be <u>something</u> more comfortable than the one I've been using. Talked to the store's owner, a fortyish, tanned, lean cyclist, who told me how to find the Verizon store and gave me directions to get to the city's western side and from there to Cañon City. He assured me I would be able to cross the Rockies. By the time I finished at the bike shop, rode across the city, went to a Verizon store to see about the problem with my cell phone, and found a Super 8 motel on US 50, it was 3 pm and 100°, hot by any standard.

62 miles = 2,208

A brief word on bicycle shops. I had tried twice and failed to fill the bike's tires at gas stations when I was training. As a result I concluded, mistakenly, as I later learned, that I shouldn't do it, for fear that I might blow out a tube and maybe a tire at the same time. So, along the way I stopped at bicycle shops whenever I could to have air put into the tires. I went as many as three days between bike shops and as a consequence lost some air pressure, but not so much that it seemed to slow me down. In addition to getting the tires pumped up, I sometimes needed adjustments to the brakes or gearshifts, and I received useful advice on what lay ahead. Also, it was nice to talk to shop owners or employees about their town, their cycling experiences, or other things of interest.

From the journal:

Day 42: Tuesday, June 18. For breakfast I had coffee, a candy bar, two donuts, and a banana in my room. At 6:20 I was on US Rte 50 headed for Cañon City. For the third day in a row the sky was empty of clouds. As I began to approach the western slope of the Rockies, the countryside got drier and drier. Today's ride included some steep hills, as the altitude rose 800 feet between Pueblo and Cañon City, 36 miles to the west. It was cool (59°) when I left but warmed up quickly. I made reasonably good time, the predicted headwind having lasted for just an hour, and arrived in Cañon City a few minutes after 10, by which time the temperature had already risen to 93°. Had a bite to eat at a cafe and bought Powerade and bottled water at a convenience store for tomorrow's ride, if I make it. I say "if" because again I have a leg problem. Had a cramp in my left calf last night, and the muscle remains sore today. Hope resting all afternoon and tonight will do the trick. Having arrived so early, normally I would have had a look around town, but with the temperature climbing to 100° and a sore calf muscle, it was best that I remain at the motel. Under better conditions, I would have been sorely tempted to make a 14-mile round-trip to see the spectacular Royal Gorge and the amazing bridge that spans it.

39 miles = 2,247 total

Reading this passage in my journal some years later, it is clear that I still hadn't learned the lesson of drinking enough fluids—water and sports drinks, such as Gatorade and Powerade—while riding. From Cañon City onward, I did a better job of fluid replacement and suffered no further muscle cramps on this or subsequent long-distance trips.

Back to the journal:

Day 43: Wednesday, June 19. The sky was clear, and the day promised to be warm, possibly hot. My legs seemed to be ok, and after a breakfast of (good) pancakes, I hit the road. The two miles through town were flat, as were the next two afterward. From there, for over a mile the road sloped gently upward. Then began the test I'd been told to expect—a steady, steep, hard climb that went on for three miles or so. I was in my lowest gear most of the time, riding at 4-5 mph. Would have gone faster were it not for a light headwind. The road went north, curving in a wide arc first to the west and then southwest. US 50 follows the narrow canyon carved out by the Arkansas River, and the wind, constricted by the canyon walls, takes the same direction as the canyon.

When the climb ended, the road leveled off for a bit and then went downhill rather sharply for a couple of miles. To keep from going too fast, I kept touching the brakes. Thirty-four miles from Cañon City, at 10:25 I came to the tiny town of Cotopaxi, where I stopped at a café for a second breakfast. Five miles later, the canyon opened to a valley that extended a few miles to the west and about twice that distance to the north. As I entered the valley, the wind velocity, which had increased to about 15 mph, decreased, and I realized, drawing on my navy training in meteorology, that I was experiencing an example of the "funnel effect." Without going into the physics of the Bernoulli Principle, this is a phenomenon that occurs when a wind hits a mountain barrier and the barrier is broken by a pass, in this case the opening to the canyon, causing the air to be forced through with considerable velocity. So in a reversal of this, when I came out of the canyon into the relatively wide valley, the wind speed dropped.

After several miles, the valley narrowed into a canyon again and once more the road ran right by the river, following its northwest course to Salida. The canyon, with its high, rocky walls, and the river, its crystalline water sometimes rushing and creating lots of white water, was a lovely sight. Watched some river rafters hurtle by. Arrived in Salida (elevation 7,000 feet) at 1:20 pm and, because it has a

*restaurant close by, picked a Best Western from among the many mo-
tels. Weather is cooler today at this higher altitude (max. temp. 81°).*

*Yesterday, on Rte 50, I traveled on a divided highway all the way
from Pueblo to Cañon City. Today the highway was just two lanes
but had a decent asphalt shoulder except for about ten miles after
Cotopaxi, when the shoulder all but disappeared, making the riding
a bit tricky at times. I'll continue to be on Rte 50 until I get to Grand
Junction.*

60 miles = 2,307 total

The route I had chosen, more or less through the middle of the
country into and across Kansas on the way to San Francisco, had
given me essentially two choices for getting over the Continental
Divide. One was the way I was going, through Pueblo, Cañon
City, and Salida over Monarch Pass. The other choice would have
taken me on a more northerly course, entering Colorado west of
Denver. I decided against going this way for two reasons. First,
motels with nearby eating places on east-west roads in northern
Kansas, such as US 36 and US 24, would probably be scarcer
than what I would find along US 56 and Kansas Rte 96. Second,
to get to the Divide by coming from east of Denver would require
making my way through the traffic-congested metropolitan area
and then, to reach and cross Loveland Pass, hopping onto and off
I-70, only portions of which are open to bicycles. The difficulties posed by the Denver-Grand Junction route may explain why
none of the cross-country itineraries of the bicycle tours I looked

up on the Internet went that way. All things considered, although the more southerly course through Pueblo meant that I would have to ride north in Utah from Green River to Salt Lake City before heading west again for San Francisco, clearly this route was the better choice for crossing the Rocky Mountains.

Whether or not I would have the stamina needed to ride a bicycle over a mountain pass higher than 11,000 feet had been one of my primary concerns from the moment that I had begun planning this trip. When I had climbed Mount Kilimanjaro in 1987, the thin atmosphere of 10,000 feet and above had given me occasional throbbing headaches, and above 15,000 feet my breathing became labored. And that had been when I was 15 years younger.

As a person ages, the lungs become less elastic. The number of air sacs (alveoli) decreases, and there is a corresponding decrease in the capillaries of the lungs. The result is a reduction in the amount of oxygen diffusing from the alveoli into the blood; muscles are fueled, so to speak, less efficiently. On top of this, respiratory muscles weaken and the chest wall becomes stiffer, less able to stretch for breathing. Consequently, older people tend to have a decreased capacity for exercise.

Sounds bad, but as with other bodily changes this one needn't be all that limiting. Although regular exercise does not change the condition of the lungs and thereby increase lung capacity, it does improve the functioning of the cardiovascular system, which, in turn, more quickly and efficiently moves blood to the lungs, where it is oxygenated and then moves onward as fuel for the muscles. Because a regular exerciser's body is much more proficient at transporting and utilizing oxygen, he or she will find physical activities, such as climbing stairs, far less strenuous than a person who does not exercise.

Still, recalling Kilimanjaro and figuring that the intervening years had to have had a negative effect on my physical condition, I became almost obsessive about reducing the weight of the load I was carrying. As I have written, early on I got rid of my tent and camping gear. Later I sent home my sleeping bag, even though it provided me with an out if I ever ended up with no place to spend the night. And I kept my clothing items to an absolute minimum. Knowing I wouldn't use an entire bottle of shampoo on the trip, I had emptied half of it out before I had started riding. Every now and then I mailed home the maps and credit card receipts that I no longer needed. Even though I came to have no doubt that I would reach the summit at Monarch Pass, I still was not sure that I would be able to pedal all the way to the top, that I would not have to walk part of the time.

From the journal:

Day 44: Thursday, June 20. Salida. Stayed the day here to be sure I'll be fresh for tomorrow's climb. Rode into town this morning to mail photos to Julie. Salida has an attractive downtown with many Victorian buildings and it appeals to tourists and people who come to fish, hike, river raft or otherwise take advantage of the town's beautiful surroundings. I visited Salida's library, its bookstore, and one of its bike shops. The shop's owner assured me that I could manage the climb to the top of Monarch Pass, but I remain a bit anxious about the combination of a long climb to the pass, especially the last several miles, which are said to be formidable, and the 11,312-foot altitude. He also told me that US 50 between Cañon City and Salida, my route yesterday, is the most dangerous road for cycling in Colorado. Just as well I didn't know that beforehand. The temperature today remained in the 70s, and the wind blew all day from the east.

Day 45: Friday, June 21. The east wind had turned to the southwest this morning when I left Salida at 6:15; so much for the pleasing prospect of an easterly tailwind. Nevertheless the wind was not much of a factor during the climb. At Poncha Springs, five miles up the road, I had breakfast. Eight miles later, I had to surmount a 1¼-mile steep grade. Less than a mile afterward, another steep climb, this one for 1.1 miles. Next, at 9:15, came the more than six-mile steady ascension to the Monarch Pass summit. For most of this, I stayed in my lowest gear, rarely making more than 4 mph. But despite the earlier climbs this morning, I was feeling in good shape, apparently not affected by the altitude, and was now confident that I'd make it to the top under my own steam without dismounting. The road went up past stands of evergreen trees, occasional meadows, rock cliffs, an old mining site, and the Monarch ski resort. I chanced upon a black bear climbing up to the roadside; he scooted away when he saw me.

When I reached the summit, at 10:40, the place was crowded with dozens of cyclists and more were arriving from the west. They and the many more I would pass as I rode down from the summit comprise the 2,000 people who are participating in the annual "Ride the Rockies" tour this year. Those I talked with said they started and will finish at Alamosa. Because their fee included transport of baggage, limited to one bag, they were not burdened with packed saddlebags, which made me stand out and led to questions about my

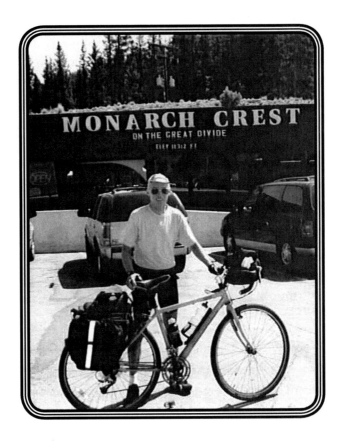

ride. After the conversations and getting my picture taken in front of the summit sign, I headed down the other side of the Continental Divide, coasting for ten miles. Great, just great! At a small town called Sargents, I stopped for a hamburger and a beer and, before continuing on, talked to some more cyclists who were heading up the pass. For much of the way from there to Gunnison the road sloped gradually downward, and despite a headwind for much of the way, I made good time. The last ten miles to Gunnison were not easy, however, as there were some hills to get over. I got into Gunnison (elevation 7,700 feet) around 2:20. With similar-looking, attractive downtowns, both Gunnison and Salida have populations of about 5,500 and cater to tourists and visitors who come to enjoy outdoor activities. I rode around town, bought a pair of riding shorts at a bicycle store, and got Powerade and water for tomorrow.

66 miles = 2,373 total

I guess you could say that this day I had a Rocky Mountain high or, an even worse pun, that I was on top of the world. But make no mistake about it, even though there was nothing remarkable about what I had accomplished, I was more than pleased to have done it. My concerns about the combination of age and altitude had proven unwarranted. Because I had been gradually gaining in altitude for the past two weeks, my body was well acclimated to the thinner air. And by now my cycling muscles were in good shape. More than likely I needn't have bothered to take the day off in Salida.

I knew there would be some tough days ahead before I got to San Francisco but figured that, having crossed the Continental Divide without trouble, I could handle whatever was ahead of me. My next test would come right away. Although I had gotten over the Divide, I was still in the Sawatch Range of the Rockies and had some more climbing to do before reaching Montrose on my way to Grand Junction.

As I wrote in the journal, I had a beer with lunch at Sargents. Also had one with lunch back in Illinois. Some might disapprove of drinking even just one beer while riding a bicycle. In theory I can agree because alcohol does slow one's reflexes. However, in practice one beer with a meal had no noticeable effect on me.

Day 46: Saturday, June 22. Because there would be no place to get food for many miles, before leaving Gunnison I waited until a restaurant across the highway from the motel opened at 6 am. It was nice to have a tailwind, only a slight one, but a tailwind nevertheless. After one hour I'd gone 15 miles. Although some inclines slowed me up, over the next hour I added on another 12 miles. US 50 passed through some impressive mountain scenery, including the Blue Mesa, and alongside it, the Blue Mesa Reservoir.

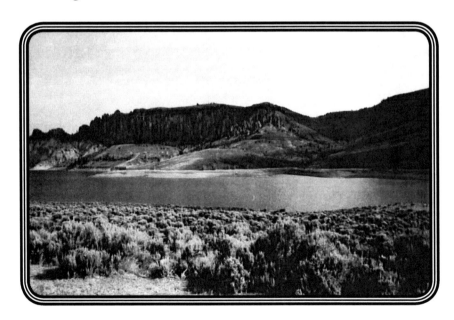

From about mile 27, I began the first of three steep, long ascents. Here the road rose 1,000 feet, from 7,500 to 8,500 feet. It seemed to me that the steepness was more pronounced than the grade on the east side of Monarch Pass, but perhaps it was just that my legs had been affected by yesterday's ride. After this first climb came a two-mile fast descent that was followed almost immediately by another formidable ascent, from 8,000 to 8,700 feet. For both climbs, I had to work fairly hard to maintain 4 mph. The welcome descent from the second one lasted for a euphoric four and a half miles. At its end and just before the beginning of the next climb, I stopped at a café at Cimarron for a hamburger. The café, a small rock shop, and a general store with two gas pumps seem to be all there is to Cimarron, or at least all I could see.

So far, the day had gone well. But as soon as I rode out of Cimarron and began the last big climb of today's ride, a west wind began blowing with a vengeance, at times gusting so hard that I was momentarily forced to a complete stop. I struggled to keep going at 4 mph but twice had to get off and walk for a few minutes.

Finally, some 15 miles east of Montrose, I crested the summit and started down into a wind that blew even harder, reducing my speed considerably, and even though still going downhill, I had to pedal hard now and then to keep going. This gale-force wind was as strong as any I have experienced on the entire trip, and I was relieved to arrive in Montrose and get a room at the Red Barn Hotel at 2:30.

66 miles = 2,439 total

I would learn later that the wind in Montrose that day gusted to 36 mph. On the Beaufort scale, winds from 31-38 mph are classified as moderate gales.

The descent from Monarch Pass to Gunnison ate up about 4,000 feet of altitude and the road dropped another 2,000 feet from Gunnison to Montrose (elevation 5,806 feet). But as my journal shows, far from going steadily downward, the descent was interrupted several times by upward slopes. The overall lower elevations brought a change in scenery, as the evergreen forests thinned out then gave way to more open spaces. Throughout those two days, every twist and turn of the road afforded picture-postcard vistas, made all the more enjoyable by the very low volume of traffic.

By the time I reached the 20-mile-long Blue Mesa Reservoir, 19 miles west of Gunnison, trees had all but disappeared and sagebrush extended from the road to the reservoir's shoreline. "Reservoir" doesn't do justice to the man-made lake, Colorado's largest body of water, created when in 1965 a dam was built on the Gunnison River. US 50 runs along its northern bank for most of its length, crossing to the southern side on a bridge at a narrow part of the reservoir about six miles from its western terminus. Closer to Montrose the hills became barer, but the landscape was softened by tall green grasses covering the flat areas between the road and the hills.

The two hours I took to pass by the Blue Mesa reservoir, stopping occasionally to appreciate the beauty of the surroundings, constituted one of those times that both defined and underlined the pleasures of riding across the country. This part of the trip manifested again that a slow passage through the United States by bicycle is sometimes rewarded by a vista of extraordinary beauty.

From the journal;

Day 47: Sunday, June 23. It was dark when I left this morning at 5:15. Rode two miles to a truck stop café, which opened at 5:30. After breakfast, I was on my way at 6:15, still on US 50. With no wind and no hills, I rode 17 miles in the next hour. Shortly afterward I stopped in the small town of Delta to buy another disposable camera. Four miles later a bug flew into my left eye, causing so much irritation that after a few minutes I had to stop and apply eye drops. Then came some rises, slowing me down, not much at first but more

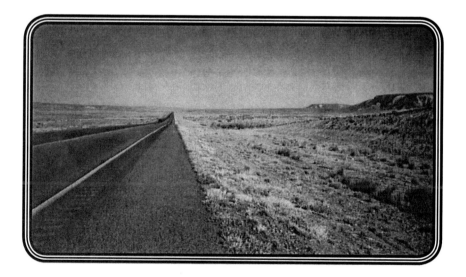

Lonesome road, Montrose to Grand Junction

so as they became steeper. Several required the granny gear and more exertion than I would have chosen to make in the intensifying heat of the day. At 9:30, after an especially tough ascent, I was rewarded with an enjoyable downhill and, at the same time, the sudden onset of a tailwind. Even after the road leveled off, I was able to sail along at 20 mph in what seemed to me almost like a dream as, pushed by the wind, I needed to pedal only occasionally.

Then, as suddenly as it had begun, the wind vanished, leaving me to deal with a few more hills several miles from Grand Junction, which I reached at 11:20. I rode another three miles to a motel on the northwestern side of the city. All in all, a very good ride today.

64 miles = 2,503 total

Now well clear of the Rockies, on this day I had reached the eastern limit of the Colorado Plateau, an area located mainly in Utah but also in parts of Colorado, New Mexico, and Arizona. Sandwiched between the Great Basin to the west and the Rockies to the east, the Plateau includes a variegated landscape of mountains, broad plateaus, and deeply eroded canyons.

Following the course of the Gunnison River Valley, US 50 took me through countryside that became increasingly arid as I made my way west to Grand Junction. From now until I began climbing the Sierra Nevada Mountains, I would be passing through the Great Basin Desert, a land often desolate but always beautiful.

CHAPTER 9

Utah

Some people have analysis. I have Utah.

Robert Redford

I grew up in Ireland, and the ocean was never more than an arm's length away. As lovely as the mountains are and as friendly as the people of Utah are, I feel a bit landlocked there from time to time.

Roma Downey

I had yet to accomplish a "century." However, I was about to leave Grand Junction bound for Green River, Utah, and because between the two towns there would be no place to stay, or even to eat, I had no option but to cover the 100 or so miles in one day.

To get to Green River, I would ride on I-70. Until now, the only time I had had access to an interstate highway was when I crossed the Mississippi River. Colorado, Utah, and Nevada are among the states that permit bicycle use of interstate highways when no feasible alternate route exists, which is the situation between Grand Junction and Green River.

Riding a bicycle on an interstate in many places might be unnerving because of a heavy volume of high-speed traffic—think of Los Angeles. But in Utah and Nevada cycling on interstates is a different proposition because generally traffic on the two interstates I used, I-70 and I-80, is not heavy. In fact, I learned by experience that there are three advantages for using an interstate. First, the wonderfully wide, well maintained road shoulders. A cyclist can ride well to the right of the roadway, putting a lot of space between rider and motor vehicles. Second, interstates are divided highways, which means there will be no problem arising from oncoming traffic. And third, as a rule interstates tend to have less steep inclines than other highways.

From the journal:

Day 48: Monday, June 24. I knew that Green River, Utah, is about 100 miles from Grand Junction and that, on the road between the two, there is no possibility of obtaining food or lodging. With that in mind, I commenced riding at 4:22 am, which was as early as I could manage. For breakfast I had coffee and two high-carb pastries, a banana, and fresh orange juice, all of which, except the coffee, I bought the previous afternoon at a supermarket. US 50, here a four-lane divided highway, is well lighted for several miles, but when I left the outskirts of Grand Junction, the roadway was dark. I could see the white lines marking the lanes but, since I foolishly had not equipped the bike with a headlight, nothing in the lanes themselves or in the shoulder, and I worried that I could run into a big pothole or something lying in the road. However, I was lucky, and not long after I had turned onto Interstate 70, the onset of daylight made the road surface fully visible.

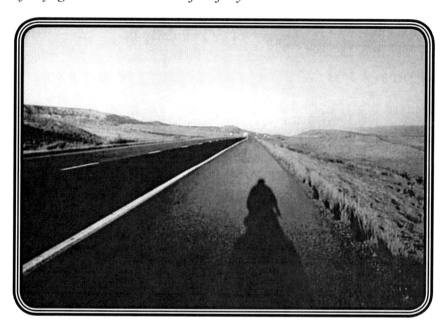

For a while the starkly beautiful semi-desert country I passed through was like a shallow Grand Canyon, with buttes and mountains sculpted by ancient streams.

After I was well clear of Grand Junction the temperature dropped so much that I had to stop to put on more clothing. By 7:30, however, it was warm enough for me to remove the extra layer, and by mid-morning it was hot, well into the 80s. By the time I arrived in Green River, the temperature had risen to 97°. From 8 until noon an easterly wind blew, softly at first but at times reaching 10-15 mph, which, together with an absence of any significant hills, allowed me to make such good time that I reached Green River, 101 miles from my starting point, at 12:30. I was jubilant for having ridden my first century. One mile later I checked into a motel. Seems odd that my legs, which have had fatigue problems as recently as yesterday, are fine after today's long, hot ride. Perhaps the hot baths, stretching, and massage have done some good.

102 miles = 2,605 total

The Green River, the largest tributary of the Colorado River, flows south from Wyoming, reaching the Colorado south of Moab near Lake Powell. After lunch, I rode through the small town of Green River (pop. about 900) and stopped to visit the John Wesley Powell River History Museum. Among its exhibits were materials relevant to the expedition Powell led in 1869 down the full extent of the Green to the confluence with the Colorado. From there Powell and the other five men who had not left the expedition, as four had, became the first non-native Americans to pass through the Grand Canyon. Gazing over the sun drenched, arid expanse of semi-desert, I could only marvel at the courage and tenacity of Powell and his men.

I felt good about having ridden the century only a few days after crossing the Rockies. With San Francisco now only about a couple of weeks away, I began to allow myself to envisage riding onto and across the Golden Gate. The next day, however, my cross-country ride came a cropper.

Day 49: Tuesday, June 25. Couldn't leave Green River early. With no source of food between there and Wellington, 57 miles to the north, I had to wait until the restaurant adjacent to the motel opened at 6. I pulled out of town at 7. For the first day in a week, there were clouds in the sky, mainly some cirrus, but they were too sparse to keep the temperature from reaching almost 100° later in the day. Despite a moderate headwind, I managed to make 19 miles by 9, when it died down, and I picked up speed for the next hour or so. However, a steep, long climb to the top a ridge at mile 37 and the intensifying heat began to take a toll on me, and I began to wonder if I could make it to Price, 65 miles from Green River. From then on, though, there were no more upward inclines, and, buoyed by the easier going, I reached Wellington at around 1. What a difference a day makes. Yesterday, after six hours I had ridden 75 miles and was showing no signs of fatigue. In the same span of time today, I had gone only 57 miles and was tired from my exertion and the heat. Had a sandwich and a coke at Wellington and left for Price at 1:30, revived by the food, drink, and rest and by learning that the road between Wellington and Price was flat all the way. After seven miles, I was approaching the first exit off Rte 6 into Price, riding on the shoulder of the two-lane road, as I had been all day, when, all of a sudden, wham! Not much later, I was in the emergency room of Price's Castleview Hospital.

The car that hit me, a Utah Highway Patrol officer told me, was going about 50 miles an hour when the young woman driver took her eyes off the road as she reached down to pick up a cup of coffee from the floorboard, whereupon her car swerved into the shoulder and struck my bike. I was lucky that the blow was to the left rear pannier and not my leg, a bit farther up the bike. I was also lucky that when I landed, my torso and not my head struck the ground. When I came to rest after rolling over several times, I lay motionless for a while, wondering how badly I was hurt. Then, because I felt no stabs of pain, I decided to get up. Gingerly, not wanting to aggravate any possible bone fracture, I rose to my knees and then stood upright, pleased that I seemed to be essentially intact.

Some motorists who had seen the accident and stopped came rushing up to me and asked if I wanted an ambulance. Still not feeling any pain, I assured them that I did not. Soon two Utah Highway Patrol officers arrived on the scene, and about the same time the car that had hit me retuned. The young woman had kept going until stopped by a man who had followed her after witnessing the accident. She had kept on going, she told him and later the police, because she thought that, from the sound of the impact, that she had hit a cardboard box, not someone on a bicycle. One of the patrolmen said he had seen me a couple of miles back and had noticed how visible the bike and I were because of the fluorescent-yellow windbreaker I had tied to the rack holding the panniers. He marveled how careless she had been. Looking at her on the other side of the highway and seeing that she was distraught, I waved to indicate that I was all right, which only seemed to make her all the more upset. The next day, a highway patrolman told me she had not been charged with hit and run, but just with driving into a lane closed to motor vehicles. I had no problem with that.

I was bleeding from some cuts and while talking with the patrolman began feeling some pain when I tried to move my right arm. By now, worried that I might not be able to continue the journey, I agreed when he said he wanted to drive me to the hospital, and thanked the spectator who offered to take the bike in his pickup to the police station.

It didn't take the young attending physician at the emergency room of Price's Castleview Hospital long to diagnose my main injury as a broken right collarbone. After tending to the cuts and abrasions on my hands, back and legs, he wrote a prescription for painkillers and gave me both a brace and a sling for the collarbone, saying that I could use either one. He went on to tell me in no uncertain terms that there was no way I could continue riding to San Francisco. Not that I needed his admonition; the growing pain and my inability to use my right arm made it clear to me that the ride had come to an end.

This turn of events deeply disappointed me, marking as it did, an abrupt end to my quest to ride from coast to coast. But I soon got over the dejection, knowing that there was nothing I could do to alter what had happened, that I should be thankful I was still alive and not badly injured, and that I had little right to complain and should pull up my socks and get on with my life.

I called the nearby Holiday Inn, which sent a van to pick me up. The next day, with the help of Holiday Inn van's driver, I picked up the bike at the Highway Patrol office, took it to Price's bicycle shop, had it crated, and took it and the panniers with my gear to UPS for shipment home. I can't say enough about the kindness of the staff at the Holiday Inn and the driver of the van in doing all they did to help me. The following day I caught an express shuttle van to the Salt Lake City airport, and the day after that I flew home.

The break in the collarbone was clean, there were no complications, and after five weeks I was able to stop using the sling. The physician in the ER in Price had told me that a broken collarbone (clavicle) is the most commonly fractured bone of the body. It used to be thought that in falls collarbone fractures often occurred because the person falling extended an arm or both arms to break the fall, thereby transferring the force of the fall onto the clavicle. Recent medical research has shown that in fact most clavicle fractures result from a blow directly on the clavicle itself.

After a couple of months of physical therapy, I regained full use of my right arm. At first when friends asked whether I'd ride long distance again, I equivocated, not sure of what I wanted to do. But it wasn't long before I came to the conclusion that it would be a shame not to finish what I had started. I decided I would pick up where I left off in Price and ride from there to San Francisco.

Various obligations prevented me from beginning serious training until the end of summer, which meant that I would not be ready to resume the ride until well into October. Having learned that heavy snowfalls are not unusual in the Sierras as early as October, I was not surprised when people in Nevada whom I contacted advised me not to try to cross the Sierras at that time of the year. Accordingly I decided to wait until the spring of 2003.

PART II

CHAPTER 10

Basin and Range

A silent world of austere beauty, of hundreds of discrete mountain ranges that are green with junipers and often white with snow....

John McPhee

Steep climbs up elongate mountain ranges alternate with long treks across flat, dry deserts, over and over and over again!

US Geologic Service

On a clear day, you can see halfway across Nevada. And the stars? Oh, man.

John Gray

At 72 I was another year older, which meant that I would not be as fit as I was a year earlier. Or did it? If you look at age from the standpoint of decades, the passage of time definitely takes a physical toll.

All things being equal, athletes at 60 will not be able to perform at the same level they did at age 50, and at 70 less ably than at 60. The physiological changes brought about by aging ensure that this will happen. But from one year to the next, the decline can be slight.

Throughout the winter I exercised four to five and sometimes six times a week—going to spin cycling classes, running and, a few times, doing some cross-country skiing. This was pretty much the same kind and extent of training that I had done the year before. However, I added some work on my leg muscles by using weight machines, and it may have made a difference, for on the ride from Price to San Francisco I had no instances of fatigue, suffered no muscle cramps, and seemed to be fitter than I had been a year earlier.

It goes without saying that a tough regimen of exercise is necessary for an out of the ordinary physical challenge, such as strenuous competitive sports or, for that matter, riding a bike across America. A much less intense effort will suffice for maintaining or achieving good health. There is a common factor, however, and that is a disciplined approach. You should set a schedule of exercise or physical activity and do all you can to stick to it. To do otherwise is to court failure.

I could handle strenuous training. For one thing, I was motivated by a strong desire to start where I left off in Utah and finish the ride to San Francisco. But doing the weight work to strengthen my legs and also exercises to avert a recurrence of a chronic back problem was a drag. I really do not like to do repetitive sets of exercises. So it was very necessary for me to set a training schedule and stick to it, often if not always.

On May 12, I kissed Julie goodbye once again and boarded a flight bound for Salt Lake City.

From my journal:

May 13. Arrived in Price at 3 pm after a two-hour drive from the Salt Lake City airport in a van. I had brought with me as accompanied baggage my bike (in a box) and panniers and riding gear (in a suitcase). Checked into the Holiday Inn, where I had stayed last year and, once again driven in the motel's van, took the bike to Decker's Bicycle Shop to have it reassembled. Picked it up at 5 and went for a ride. Rode south of town to US Rte 6 and, recognizing the manhole cover I had rolled next to, I stopped and dismounted at the exact spot where I had been hit. Disappointed that the good people of Price and not erected a statue in my honor, I rode back through town to the motel. My plan is to stay here until I'm acclimated to the 5,000-foot altitude.

Wednesday, May 14. Trial run this morning. Rode 16 miles from Price in a northwesterly direction on Rte 6. The climb to Soldier Summit begins just beyond the small town of Helper, seven miles from the Holiday Inn. Because I coped well with the uphill portion of today's ride and seemed unaffected by the altitude, I decided to cut short my stay in Price and leave tomorrow. There is one motel in Helper (pop. about 2,000), a funky place called the Riverside Motel, where I reserved a room before heading back to Price. Took the suitcase and some clothing to a UPS store for shipment, checked out of the Holiday Inn, rode to Helper, and checked in at the Riverside ($31).

Riding from the motel's office to my room, I discovered that the rear tire was flat. Doggone it—Utah seemed to have it in for me. Took off the rear wheel to change the tube only to find that the spare tube (carelessly, I had brought only one) was shot. Removed the wheel and hitched a ride, in a new Cadillac, no less, to Decker's. A thorn had punctured the tire and tube. Because the tire was worn, I bought a new one along with two tubes, one of which I got installed with the tire onto the wheel. The store's friendly owner gave me a ride back to Helper, where I spent a quiet evening watching a ballgame and reading.

Helper got its name from the "helper" engines that, beginning in the latter part of the nineteenth century, were added there to the Denver and Rio Grande Western Railway trains that needed more power to carry cars laden with coal from nearby mines. The coal cars had to be hauled up the steep 15-mile climb northwestward through Price Canyon to Soldier Summit on the way north to Salt Lake City and beyond. As I set out to begin the ascent from Helper, the view was daunting—an almost vertical barren ridge rising a few hundred feet directly north of the town.

From the journal:

Thursday, May 15. Day one of this part of the renewed journey, or day 50 of the total NH-to-San Francisco trip. Beginning mileage is 2,680, which includes last year's total of 2,669 miles, plus the four from the spot of the accident to the motel in Price and the seven from Price to Helper.

At about 7, after eating a sandwich and a Snickers bar and downing a cup of coffee at the convenience store across the highway from the motel, I departed Helper in a steady light rain that continued for the next two hours. Two miles beyond the town, I began the ascent to Soldier Summit, which at times had a steep gradient.

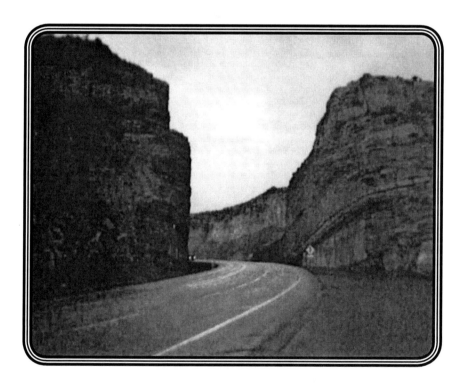

A light headwind wasn't much of a problem at first, and I averaged about 7 mph during the 3 hours and 20 minutes it took me to reach the summit. About a half-hour out of Helper I stopped for a drink, only to discover I'd left my bottles of Gatorade and water in

the motel room. Aargh! The cool (low 40s), moist weather helped keep my thirst in check, but a couple of times I was thirsty enough to resort to licking the accumulated water on my windbreaker sleeves. Came upon a small general store an hour north of the summit and bought water and Gatorade. At the summit I zoomed down for about 11 miles. Near the end of the descent the wind became strong, and the next 20 miles, even though most of it was slightly downhill, required a fair amount of pedal power.

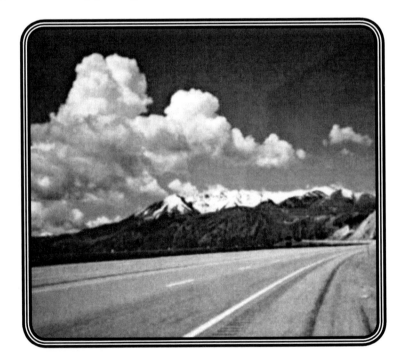

South of Provo

This part of US 6 was a mixed bag. Sometimes the shoulder was a generous three feet or more and at other times extremely narrow. Traffic was moderate today, but much of it consisted of trucks, which, when there wasn't much of a shoulder, came unpleasantly close to me now and then. Was I conscious that the accidental death insurance policy I bought for the trip won't take effect until tomorrow? Yep. Fifty-eight miles from Helper I came to Utah Rte 89, which I took to Provo, passing through a couple of towns on the way, relieved that there was less traffic and the wind was no long blowing at me. Had lunch at a Subway around 2:00, then rode on to Provo, where I got directions to local motels. Checked into a Holiday Inn around 3:30.

Today was a good start, I'd say. I passed the altitude test in good shape, arriving in Provo tired but nowhere near exhausted.

70 miles = 2,750 total

Again demonstrating that I was in pretty good shape, the climb from Helper, elevation 5,830, to Soldier Summit, 7,477 feet, did not take much out of me. No one lives in the abandoned town that once housed or catered to three hundred inhabitants. Dilapidated weather-beaten structures—mainly a few deserted houses—some crumbling walls, and acres of foundations are all that remains of the town of Soldier Summit, which has the official status of a Utah ghost town.

By now I had ridden all but a few miles of the 132-mile length of US Highway 6. Extending from Green River to Spanish Fork, several miles south of Provo, US 6 has a justly earned reputation, based on fatal accidents, as Utah's most dangerous highway. Ironically, the portion of US 6 going into Price where I was hit by a car is not considered dangerous at all. As for the road between

Price and the turnoff to Provo, I believe the danger is more to cars than to bicycles. There were moments, as I noted in the journal, when narrow roadway shoulders didn't provide much space between passing trucks and me. But this was no worse than what I had experienced on some other roads in other states, Missouri for example. Still, it affirmed the need to concentrate on keeping as far to the right as possible and the wisdom of keeping the upper body clad in very bright, easily visible clothing.

There is a widespread perception that bicycling is an extremely dangerous activity. Is it dangerous? Sure, but so too are driving a car, skiing, snowmobiling, or even walking by a roadside, none of which is tagged as *extremely* dangerous.

In 2010, according to the US Department of Transportation 623 bicycle riders were killed in the United States. In that same year automobile accidents killed 32,788 drivers or their passengers, 4,376 motorcyclists lost their lives, and 4,280 pedestrians died after being struck by motor vehicles. These grim figures by themselves do not prove that riding a bike is safer than riding in a motor vehicle, because they do not take into consideration the miles ridden. Studies that have factored in miles ridden have presented differing conclusions as to the relative danger of motoring, cycling, or walking along roadways. So the answer as to how dangerous or how safe cycling is has to be that there is no conclusive proof one way or the other. But it is quite likely that the widespread perception that cycling is very dangerous is not likely to be erased.

Bicycle riding would be safer than it is if more people wore helmets, inasmuch as statistics demonstrate that helmets are effective in reducing head and brain injuries. I wasn't wearing a helmet when I flew through the air after being hit by a car in Utah. Luckily, I didn't land on my head or hit something head-first. Months later, when I resumed riding, I wore a helmet except sometimes when climbing at a snail's pace (which I have to admit was not too smart, for, as one of my daughters pointed out to me, after being hit by a car a bike rider could be flying at a fast rate when striking the ground or some stationary object).

From the journal:

Day 2 (51 of the total ride). Friday, May 16. Another 7 am departure. Clear and not as cold as yesterday. Went west for a few miles, then north and northwest on Utah Rte 114. Passed through an industrial area and then a collection of second-rate strip malls and the usual assortment of fast-food joints, gas stations, body shops, etc. What a contrast between this and the beautiful snow-capped mountain ranges that sandwich the valley leading up to Salt Lake.

The route I followed avoided, for a while, the heavy traffic on the valley floor, but before long the traffic thickened and I got off Rte 114 and rode farther west to Utah 68, which begins in a rural area and proceeds north a couple hundred feet above the valley, passing over slopes leading upward toward the mountain range on my left. By about 30 miles from my start at Provo, the surroundings had segued from rural to suburban to urban, and Rte 68 had widened from a two-lane road with no shoulder, which made for some uncomfortable moments, to six-lanes. As the traffic became heavier, when no people were walking on sidewalks I rode on them because often motorists weren't giving me much leeway. At 12:20, a couple of miles or so east of the heart of Salt Lake City's downtown, I came to I-80, which runs east-west, rode under it, and proceeded a block farther north, where I found a Holiday Inn, a convenience store, and some restaurants. Bought bananas and Gatorade for tomorrow, checked into the motel, had lunch, and called it a day.

51 miles = 2,801 total. This trip = 121

Ahead of me lay the Great Salt Lake Desert, which extends from just west of Salt Lake City to Wendover at the Nevada line. Although earlier apprehensive about crossing this desolate stretch of land, now feeling strong and knowing the weather most probably would be favorable, I was looking forward the coming day's ride. Whatever it might bring, it would be interesting.

Day 3 (52). Saturday, May 17. Today's conditions were just about ideal for the long ride. In the 40s when I started, the temperature stayed in the 50s most of the morning. After breakfast at a Denny's, at 0545 I rode one block to the I-80 on-ramp and headed west. The darkness held for about 30 minutes. When the sky had lightened

sufficiently I turned off the flashlight I had duct-taped to the handle-bar bag. No hills for two hours, and I averaged 12 mph, a light breeze from the west and an occasional gradual upslope slowing me down only slightly. The divided highway is built on two parallel embankments, raising it above the level of the Great Salt Lake. Skirting the lake, the road passes to the north of the Oquirrah Mountains—some 15 miles or so from my starting point—and then the Stansbury Mountains, another 25 miles farther along.

Fifty miles down the road at 10:20, I reached Delle, which is not a town as such, just a gas station, a long-abandoned motel and, making my morning, the Skull Valley Café, where I had another breakfast and used the bathroom. When I exited the café, I found that a fresh breeze from the northwest had begun to blow. Since at this point I-80 turns from west to northwest, I would have to contend with a headwind. Using more effort than I wanted to exert, I managed to average 6 or 7 mph. Fortunately, after 8 miles the highway angled to the southwest, and wind was no longer a factor. Several miles farther along I came to the only rise of any consequence between Salt Lake and Wendover. The half-mile climb there was more than compensated by a two-mile descent. A high overcast kept the day cool well into the afternoon, and the high temperature for the day would only be 72°. Cars, trucks, and motorcycles zoomed by me at speeds, for the most part, well over the posted limit of 75 mph. But the shoulder was wide and, except for a 20-mile stretch, in good condition.

Now the desert country took on a fascinating barren cast, with Lake Desert to the south (on my left) and Evaporation Basin to the north beginning at about mile 90. My legs were getting a little tired, but I knew I'd make it to Wendover. There was just one problem—It had been four hours since I left Delle and I had to go. Unfortunately, for mile after mile there was nothing more along the road than foot-high spindly plants, no place for the cover my modesty demanded. Then, far ahead I could see a structure of some kind. With increasing urgency I pedaled and pedaled, finally reaching a 50-foot high column surmounted by multi-colored large spheres. A 20-yard dirt path led from the highway to the sculpture's column, whose diameter was more than ample enough to screen me. Ah, relief! On a small plaque on the column, I read, "Metaphor: The Tree of Utah".

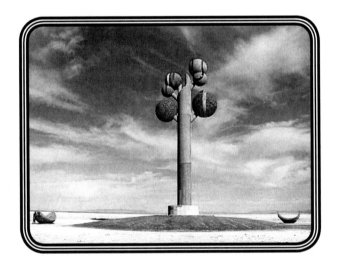

This is an appropriate place to note that the majority of men age 60 and above, as many as 80 percent, experience some sort of problem with urinating due to prostate enlargement. It's also noteworthy that regular exercise reduces moderate and severe symptoms of the enlargement. And there is evidence that men over 65 who regularly exercise have as much as a 70 percent lower risk of being diagnosed with advanced prostate cancer. It is not clear, though, whether it is the exercise itself that causes the lower incidence of prostate cancer or because the regular exercisers' overall health makes them less susceptible to the disease. For example, they would be much less likely to be obese, and there is a known link between obesity and prostate cancer.

Given that I was riding for up to ten hours a day, I had reason to be thankful that the extent of my prostate enlargement, whatever it might have been, was not so much as to cause me have to make frequent pit stops.

Back to the journal:

After 100 miles, the intensity of the pristine whiteness of the salt flats was extraordinary. I made good time over the next 20 or so miles, skipped the exit to Wendover, Utah, and rode on to the next one, the exit to West Wendover, Nevada. Having heard that casino/hotels on the Nevada side have low fares as a lure for gamblers, I was disappointed to find that the prices are steeply hiked up on weekends. Told at the first one I entered that I'd have to pay $100 for a room and that there were no non-smoking rooms, I got back on the bike and rode to the Utah side of town. Lots of motels at reasonable prices but no nearby restaurants. So back I went to Nevada. Just across the line, the Montego Bay offered a non-smoking room for $70, and I checked in around 5 o'clock. A long day, but I was happy to have ridden 125 miles.

125 miles = 2,926 total. This trip = 246

From the time that I had decided on the route I would take to get from Utah to San Francisco, I had been uneasy about the Salt Lake City-Wendover leg of the journey, worried that a combination of headwinds and high temperatures could find me in the desert with not enough energy to make the rest of the way to Wendover on my own. It was clear to me, though, that I had little choice but to go that way.

As it happened, I managed the ride between Salt Lake City and West Wendover handily. It could have been a different story if I had not had the accident in Price and had set out from Salt Lake City as I had intended on June 27, 2002, a day during which the temperature rose to 99 degrees. But chances are that with a very early start well before sunrise, I could have made it to Wendover all right, since on that day there were no adverse winds to buck. Much of the rest of the trip across Nevada would have been problematical, however, because the combination of winds and temperatures I would have faced would have been intimidating, to put it mildly. Available historical meteorological data show that the high heat and strong headwinds I would have run into in Nevada would have been formidable. The temperature reached 98 degrees between Wendover and Wells, with a headwind gusting to 32 mph, and conditions were almost identical on the succeeding five days until Fernley, the last stop before Carson City. Traveling now in the spring instead of the summer and being much luckier with the winds, I had an easier time of it.

There is an alternative route through Nevada, US Rte 50. However, to have reached it from Green River, instead of riding north to Salt Lake City I would have had to continue riding west on I-70 from Green River for 103 miles over semi-desert terrain to the small town of Salina, with not so much as a gas station in between. At Salina, I-70 intersects US 50, which 71 uninhabited miles later, comes to Delta, the last chance in Utah to get a place to stay. Some 90 sparsely settled miles to the west of Delta, US 50 crosses into Nevada. Running more or less parallel to and about 100 miles south of I-80, US 50 features long expanses in which there are no sources of water, food, or accommodations. For me, trying to cross Nevada on US 50 would not necessarily have been suicidal, but it surely would have been foolhardy. Not for nothing is US 50 in Nevada called "The Loneliest Road in America."

From the journal:

Day 4 (53): Sunday, May 18. When I got up at 5:30 this morning and looked outside my window, I could see that the wind was blowing strongly. According to the Weather Channel, this part of Nevada will have a 20 mph northerly wind, gusting to 30 mph today and tonight. That, coupled with a sore right knee that needed icing, convinced me to spend the day here in West Wendover. Except for a walk to a convenience store to get Gatorade, water and energy bars, I have remained in the hotel. Food in the coffee shop in the casino is okay. Good news—today's room rates are back to the usual rate, $29.95. Yesterday and again today the desk clerk gave me a coupon, good for a dollar in nickels. It took me no time at all to lose the $2.00 playing the video slot machines. Then I invested $1.50 of my own money to play a blackjack machine. Same result. I wandered around *watching people gambling, most of them playing the slots, some of them intently, some with grim looks on their faces. I don't understand the attraction.*

A brief word on joints—not gambling joints, body joints. For many people, perhaps most, a conspicuous early sign of aging is stiffness. As the years go by, tendons and ligaments lose elasticity. The synovial fluid that lubricates joints decreases in amount, causing them to become stiffer and less flexible. Lack of exercise intensifies stiffness. Cartilage cushioning the joints begins to break down, causing friction between bones, further limiting mobility. Calcification can take place as minerals build up in some joints. Add to this that, according to the Center for Disease Control, 50 percent of persons ages 65 or older have medically-diagnosed arthritis.

Although all this sounds dreary, it need not be excessively limiting, because exercise can pay large dividends. Certain forms of exercise may not be possible for the older person. In particular, knee problems rule out running for many; but for the majority, jogging or running *is* possible. And contrary to popular belief, research has proved that running does not cause osteoarthritis in those with normal, uninjured knees. The Arthritis Foundation asserts that the stronger the muscles and tissues around your joints, the better they will be able to support and protect those joints, whereas without exercise, muscles become smaller and weaker. Bottom line, it is a lack of exercise rather than exercise that leads to or exacerbates joint problems.

For strengthening joints, the many alternatives to running include walking, swimming, and biking, either actual or stationary. It's worth noting that in recent years research—by the American Heart Association and Harvard Medical School, among others—has determined that walking is just as good an exercise for cardiovascular fitness as running. While running is more effective for losing weight, walking has about the same effect as running in reducing risk for high blood pressure, high cholesterol levels, and diabetes as long as runners and walkers cover the same distance and thereby expend the same amount of energy. To do this, obviously a walker will have to spend more time walking than the runner will spend running.

My specific problem, the sore knee that bothered me this day, is called "runner's knee," an irritation of the undersurface of the kneecap, which, as many cyclists can attest, is an ailment not limited to runners. A common cause of this knee pain is overuse, which for cyclists stems from excessive bending and straightening of the knee in a given period of time. My long ride from Salt Lake City to West Wendover had resulted in knee pain. Fortunately it was not severe and responded well to icing and the day of rest.

From the journal:

Day 5 (54). Monday, May 19. Although I was up before 5, I saw no need to get an early, pre-dawn start. The strong northwest wind has diminished and is forecast to shift later this morning to east-northeast. It's 39° and the maximum temperature is expected to be only 57°, a good weather day for cycling. During breakfast in the coffee shop I talked with the manager, a woman of about my age, with whom I had had a brief conversation the day before. Then and again this morning she praised me for making the journey and told me of her own adventures flying in hot air balloons and an ultralight aircraft. When I finished eating and asked for the check, she said my meal was on the house and wished me a safe and successful trip.

Left West Wendover at 7:15. Crystal-clear sky. Began with a moderately steep climb, made somewhat difficult by a wind coming in at me from a 45-degree angle on my right. The incline ended after 2 1/2 miles, and the road remained generally level for most of the next dozen miles. At about 14 miles, when I started going up a slight incline, the wind had veered 90 degrees to my right and lost most of its force. Hallelujah! One mile later the angle of climb increased but remained moderate for the six miles to the summit, Silverzone Pass, which I reached at 9:50. At 5,955 feet, the pass is 1,500 feet higher than Wendover.

Coasted downhill for four miles. The snowcapped Pequop Mountains to my left provided a scenic backdrop to the ride. Between the highway and the mountains and also stretching to my right, sage-brush and other plants softened the semi-desert vista.

As the day progressed, the traffic—mostly trucks—decreased to a trickle. Sometimes when I stopped for a drink, no vehicles were in sight or hearing, and I could relish the absolute silence. The town of Oasis, at mile 32, consisted of several gasoline pumps and a bare-bones convenience store, where I bought a bottle of Gatorade along with two cookies and a candy bar that I devoured before getting back on the road.

The second major climb of the day began right afterward. This one, five miles up to Pequop Summit, was much steeper, and even with a slight tailwind I could only manage four mph. The subsequent downhill ride was a great relief and much fun, although cold. It would have been more fun if I could have let her rip and gone a lot faster, but as usual, to keep the fully loaded bike from wobbling, I didn't go much more than 35 mph. The steep descent lasted for five miles, then moderated, continuing for several more miles. The day's final climb, beginning at about mile 50, was a gentle slope that slowed me, but only to seven mph. After that it was downhill the rest of the way to Wells, where I arrived at 2:08, which, because I had crossed into the Pacific Time Zone after leaving Wendover, was only 1:08. Nice room for $35 at the Rest Inn. Had a beer and late lunch at the casino/bar/restaurant just across the street.

61 miles = 2,987 total. This trip = 307

By now I was well into the basin and range country. Most of Nevada consists of alternating basins—valleys whose streams do not drain to the sea— and north-south mountain ranges. If you look at a topographical map of the state from above, the impression is that the land has been irregularly raked by a huge claw, which explains why traveling east to west, across basin and range, involves climbing and descending over and over again.

Traversing this area is made easier by following the corridor formed by the Humboldt River. This is as true for the cyclist today as it was for the wagon trains heading for California and Oregon in the mid-19th century, the construction of the Central Pacific Railroad across Nevada in 1868-69, and the laying down of the US 40 in the 1920s and its later improved version, Interstate-80. Snaking its way across north-central Nevada, the Humboldt intersects I-80 some 30 miles southwest of Wells and runs from there about 200 miles to Lovelock and then farther south until it loses itself in the Humboldt Sink. More a creek than a river, the shallow Humboldt generally cannot be seen from the highway, and its effects on the land through which it passes are lost to most travelers. In some places it is beautiful, as witness an exchange between John McPhee and a geologist friend traveling with him on I-80 in the early 1980s: "The Humboldt River, blue and full, was flowing toward us, with panes of white ice at its edges, sage and green meadow beside it, and dry russet uplands rising behind. I said I thought that was lovely. He said yes, it was lovely indeed, it was one of the loveliest angular unconformities I was ever likely to see."[11] Beauty as seen first through the eyes of a writer and second through the eyes of a geologist.

Unlike US 50, I-80 cannot be called a lonely road, not with its traffic and its substantial towns every 50 miles or so. Still, as I noted in my journal, there were times when I could neither see nor hear any vehicles. Once, the complete silence was all the more impressive when it was briefly broken by a bird singing. Looking east at the valley cut by the Humboldt, I could see, in my mind's eye, emigrant wagon trains plodding across the sere, desolate land, made majestic by the snowcapped mountains in the distance.

---

11   John McPhee, *Basin and Range* (New York: Farrar, Strauss, Giroux, 1981), 88.

Day 6 (53). Tuesday, May 20.

Awake and up at 5, I hoped to get an early start, since, with the change in time zone, darkness is no longer a factor after 5:30. However, after learning that the temperature this morning is 29° and having sent my sweatshirt home from Price, I decided to wait until 7:30 before beginning to ride. When I walked to the casino for breakfast, there had been icicles on the rail fence outside the motel.

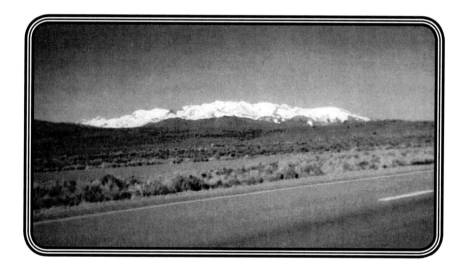

Near Wells

By the time I got underway at 7:38, the temperature was above freezing. Like yesterday, the sky was cloudless and, at Wells's altitude—5,636 feet—vividly blue.

After a two-mile gradual uphill, the road leveled off and I made good time for two hours. The rest of the way to Elko the road rose and fell as it crossed low ridges running down from the foothills of the snow-topped Humboldt Range to the south, visible on my left for the first 20 or 25 miles. The upward inclines weren't steep and the downhills were great. For three hours there was no wind, and when it began to blow, it was relatively gentle. My route today was generally to the southwest.

For five miles beginning about mile 25, I-80 was being repaired, with the result that of the two westbound lanes of the divided highway, one-and-a-half were scraped clean and too rough to ride on. Trucks and cars made their way on the remaining half lane and adjoining shoulder, leaving me with no room at all on the right side of the road. To keep vehicles from drifting over to the left and onto the roadway under construction, three-foot high, trash-can sized orange plastic barriers were placed every 20 yards or so on the left edge of the drivable half lane. So what I did was ride on a line with the barriers, edging farther out onto the half lane to my right as I reached each barrier, timing this maneuver so that there would be no cars or trucks nearby when I swerved around the barriers. This worked fine until a line of trucks approaching from behind came upon me as I was about to move to the right to avoid a barrier. I braked hard and, unable to release my shoe clamps in time, over I went, falling hard on my left side. No damage to the bike and only a couple of lacerations, as I discovered later, to my left knee. My old bones continue to hold up well.

Pulled into Elko, 50 miles from Wells, precisely at noon. After lunch at a McDonald's, I rode through town to Elko's bicycle shop, where I had the tires checked and pumped up to 75 lbs. of pressure. Then I headed for Carlin. Some 15 miles later, I came to a 2,000-foot tunnel that cuts through a mountain.

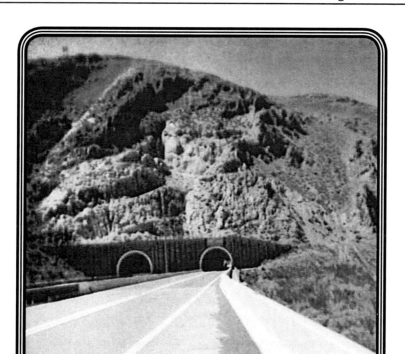

About 40 yards before the tunnel, the shoulder ends entirely and doesn't reappear until the same distance on the other side of the tunnel. That left me with no choice but to ride on the roadway until well clear of the 425 meters-long tunnel. As the owner of the bike shop in Elko had advised me, I waited until I saw no vehicles coming my way; adding to the drama, I could see only about a quarter mile back to a curve in the road. As soon as I couldn't see or hear any motor vehicle, I sprinted into the tunnel. Man, I flew, fear-induced adrenaline flowing. As I neared the end of the tunnel I could hear an increasingly load roar of an engine, which sounded loud enough to be that of truck, and I pedaled even harder. It was with great relief that

I emerged from the tunnel and moved over to the shoulder, just as a small car passed. In the confines of the tunnel, its engine noise had been greatly magnified.

At 2:30 I reached Carlin, an unprepossessing town, from what I saw of it, of some 2,000 souls. I checked in at the only motel, a Comfort Inn, just off the ramp to the highway. Looked for a restaurant, and had to settle for a Subway sandwich place. After eating, I went looking for a beer. Found a saloon/pool hall where, while I was busy with my journal, a guy asked me what I was writing. My explanation led to an invitation to play a game of 8-Ball. He wasn't very good, but I was worse. He and his companions told me that mining companies are the principal employers of Carlin's inhabitants. They said my attempt to ride to San Francisco was (what else?) "awesome." Dinner tonight was a foot-long ham sandwich at the Subway.

74 miles = 3,061 total. This trip = 381

Day 7 (56). Wednesday, May 21. The weather report this morning put Elko's temperature at 34°, which is predicted to rise to 88°, in contrast to yesterday's 72°. Since Carlin is at the same elevation, 5,000 feet, the temperature is probably the same at both towns. Breakfast consisted of two bowls of cold cereal at the motel and a ham and egg sandwich at the Subway.

Back on I-80 shortly after 6. The ascent to Emigrant Pass began about 2 ½ miles out of Carlin. For another 2 ½ miles the grade was so mild that my speed ranged between seven and 11 mph. This, I thought, was going to be a piece of cake. The upward angle increased at this point and for a mile I could go no faster than seven mph, but the climb was still easy. Then came 2.3 miles of hard work to keep going at four mph. Just shy of six miles from the beginning of the climb, the steepness eased and my speed rose to six mph. After that, another hard mile at four mph to the top.

I've put in the details because it will help me remember that this climb of eight miles from 4,959 to 6,114 feet was as demanding physically as any I have made so far since I left Price. The downhill reward was short, a little over two miles, and was followed by a half-mile climb to Twin Summit and another descent, this one for 3 ½ miles.

The highway now went up and down through rolling hills for several miles. Then from 23 miles out of Carlin on the way to Battle Mountain the roadway was more or less level as it passed over terrain through which the Humboldt River flowed. By 11 o'clock I was warm enough to strip down to shorts and T-shirt. All morning long there was only a light breeze from the south. I made good time in the valley and reached Battle Mountain by 11:40. Rode through town checking out the accommodations. I chose the Battle Mountain Inn at the town's west end and had lunch at the Broadway Colt Inn Casino, next-door. Will go back tonight for dinner and to gamble two one-dollar rolls of nickels, compliments of the motel.

52 miles = 3,113 total. This trip = 433

Wells, Elko, Carlin and Battle Mountain and also two other Nevada towns I would pass through farther west on I-80—Winnemucca, and Lovelock—were either established or given a boost when the

Central Pacific Railroad Company constructed the western portion of the first transcontinental railroad in the 1860s. Today, the economies of these towns are based on gold mining and to a lesser extent agriculture (mainly raising livestock, especially in Elko county) and gambling. Elko, the largest of northern Nevada's towns, population 17,430 in 2010, is doing better economically than the other, much smaller towns. Far removed from the large populations and glitter and growth of Las Vegas and the Reno-Sparks metropolitan area, the rural towns of northern Nevada, have their attractions but face increasing economic difficulties.

Traveling through northern Nevada accentuates the contrast between America's crowded eastern seaboard and west coast and the sparsely populated open spaces of large parts of western states. On my journey, I would ride for long periods of time during which I saw no evidence of the hand of man except for the highway and its vehicular traffic. As I slowly made my way through the empty spaces of the Great Basin's high desert, instead of bringing on a feeling of loneliness, the isolation had a certain appeal.

Day 8 (57). Thursday, May 22. Lost my $1.00 gambling stake again last night. Yesterday, after three or four hours, the ride had been so uncomfortable on my behind that before leaving this morning, I tinkered with the saddle's angle. It didn't do any good, and at 8, an hour after I left Battle Mountain following a big breakfast, I had to stop and readjust the saddle. That did the trick, and the rest of today's trip was fine.

Proceeded northwest under a clear sky as the dry weather—20 percent relative humidity—continued. No wind. Two hours and 26 miles later I reached the base of the climb to Golconda Summit. Stopped to take off my tights and windbreaker and rode off, somehow forgetting to put the tights into a pannier. Hope somebody my size will find them.

At the beginning of the ascent I managed only five mph, which presented a problem because at that slow speed I attracted flies, which, looking for breakfast, had at me. But after a mile the road leveled off for a short spell, and I left the flies behind. From there to the top, another 4 ½ miles, was no strain. Once there I put my helmet on and began a cool, relaxing four-mile downhill. Halfway down and for another three miles, thousands of crickets were traveling along the highway, the shoulder, and the arid land to my right, heading in the same direction I was going. I managed not to squish too many. A farmer would have no such compunction, for although cricket migrations are something to see, they can devastate crops.

The remainder of the approximately 15 miles to the outskirts of Winnemucca was flat except for three ridges that intersected the highway and a gradual gain in elevation for a mile or two before the East Winnemucca exit, which I reached at 11:35. Winnemucca's bicycle shop was near the center of town, three miles from the exit. The proprietor checked my tires, added a few pounds of air to each, took my picture, which he said he would email to me, and gave me advice on how to get to Carson City from Fernley. I checked into a Day's Inn ($52) and had lunch at a café across the street. Noon temperature was 82°, predicted high for the day, 90°. My legs are fine. Last night I stopped icing my right knee, and the pain in the left one, which I banged up when I fell the other day, is gone.

The scenery wasn't the greatest today, but the ride was enjoyable. This day, unlike the other days since I left Salt Lake City, there were no imposing mountain ranges in view. Winnemucca is a relatively pleasant-looking town—more spruce than the others I have passed through or stopped in since getting to Nevada. No bookstore in town, I was told, but I found something to read at a supermarket, where I also got some water, Gatorade, bananas, and sunscreen.

55 miles = 3,168 total. This ride = 488

Losing the tights wasn't the only time on the trip that I was zapped by forgetfulness. Twice, once in Ashtabula, Ohio, and once near Placerville, California, I almost lost my wallet by setting it on the rack over the bike's rear wheel and riding off before replacing it in the handlebar bag. Both times I was remarkably lucky not to lose the wallet. As I have related, In Ashtabula I heard a noise behind me as I rode away from a bicycle shop, looked back, and saw my wallet in the street. In California, I rode for four miles after leaving a convenience store near Placerville, stopping to take a banana from the handlebar bag and nearly having heart failure when I noticed the wallet was not in there. But before I even turned the bike around, I looked over my shoulder and there it was, somehow perched right where I left it on the rack. On a ride from Florida to New Hampshire a year later, I left my credit card in a restaurant, not discovering the loss for another 50 miles. Fortunately I had a spare and when I phoned the manager of the restaurant, he agreed to destroy the forgotten card.

Everyone experiences forgetfulness from time to time, some more than others, but most within a range that is perfectly normal. Forgetfulness is nothing to fret about unless it is accompanied by symptoms such as chronic lateness, frequently missed appointments, or forgotten commitments—all indications of ADD (attention deficit disorder) or possibly the onset of dementia.

According to the National Institutes of Health, the vast majority of adults do not have ADD nor do they suffer from dementia; they are simply absentminded to one degree or another. But as Americans have become more aware of the prevalence of Alzheimer's disease, many older Americans worry that their forgetfulness is a sign of the onset of some form of dementia, particularly Alzheimer's. Sad to say, it may be for some. But, again, not for most. As family and friends well know, I have been absent minded since I was young. When I was in college, much to the amusement of my roommates, I posted a note by the inside of the door of our apartment which said, "Don't forget your lunch, stupid." When I occasionally flew a light aircraft, some of my friends marveled that I didn't forget some essential procedure necessary to keep the plane in the air.

All my adult life I have spent an inordinate amount of time looking for one thing or another that I've misplaced, especially my glasses. This year I made a New Year's resolution not to lose anything of importance, like my glasses, and I've kept that resolution. Although I have *misplaced* things for as long as a few days, I haven't *lost* anything.

If forgetfulness is a normal part of the human condition, it most likely will become more pronounced as we age. So say the experts. Most people remain mentally alert, but may take longer to remember things. As aging progresses, even the healthiest of persons are less able to remember certain kinds of information. And although physical exercise can help improve mental acuity, it won't have much effect on forgetfulness.

To the long-distance rider or anyone else doing something for which a loss of an item could be disastrous, all I can say is make a conscious, major effort to focus on what you are doing. Check lists are much recommended.

Day 9 (58). Friday, May 23. Today was a mixed bag of bad luck, stupidity, good luck, and good luck again. At 6:05 I was on the road, headed for Lovelock, 72 miles southwest of Winnemucca. Passed by cattle ranches, as I did yesterday east of the town. The highway here was paved in concrete instead of asphalt. A feature of I-80—like that of many highways—is three-inch grooves about an inch deep and a foot long abutting and perpendicular to the roadway. Their purpose is to alert the motorist who drives off the highway onto the shoulder, but they jar the hell out of the careless cyclist who rides over them. Often the concrete portions of I-80 have, in addition, sets of narrower grooves that run across the full width of the shoulder and extend a yard from beginning to end. Spaced about ten yards apart, each set consists of 15 grooves. Because they are so narrow and shallow, riding over them is not unpleasant, just a gentle rumbling sensation. But they pose a potential problem because the detritus of the highway—such as sand, pebbles, and small sharp objects like shards of glass or pieces of

metal—*collects in the grooves and can damage a tire. And that's what happened to me.*

Aided by a mild tailwind, I was cruising along at 16 mph when, 9 ½ miles out of Winnemucca, the rear tire went flat. I was unlucky to have ridden over a small piece of wire, probably from the debris of a destroyed radial tire, which punctured the rear tire and tube. I took off the wheel, tire and tube, replaced the tube, put everything back together again, and put in as much air as I could with the hand pump. Ready to go again, but now I had no spare tube because, idiot that I am capable of being, I had neglected to be sure to have two spares on hand. At this point I could have gone back to Winnemucca to buy the tubes I needed. But, not wanting to add 19 miles to the day's ride, I pressed on to Lovelock.

From then on my luck was good. The grooved concrete paving of the shoulder ended after five more miles, and the rest of the way to Lovelock the shoulder was smooth and clean. And the favorable northeast wind continued much of the morning. I figured that if I couldn't find a tube in Lovelock, I'd have to hitchhike or catch a bus to Sparks, where I knew there was a bicycle shop. So I pushed myself at a faster pace than usual in order to get to Lovelock as early as I could, particularly since it was getting hot. The temperature had reached 88° by the time I reached Lovelock at 12:05, exactly 6 hours after leaving Winnemucca. I had averaged 14 mph over the 62 miles from the site of the flat tire. No bike shop in Lovelock, but a second piece of good luck—I was directed to a small hardware store, which had one tube that fit my wheel size. Checked into a Ramada Inn at 12:30.

74 miles = 3,242 total. This ride = 562

Focused as it was on the condition of the highway and the flat tire misadventure, my journal entry said next to nothing about the countryside between Winnemucca and Lovelock. The elevations of those two towns and my next-day destination, Fernley, were all in the neighborhood of 4,000 feet. Even though they were a thousand feet or more lower than the four Nevada towns I had previously passed through, they had the same physical characteristics of the basin and range semi-arid high desert. Sagebrush dominated the treeless landscape, with barren mountains in the distance to the right and left of the highway. Because of the lingering effects of fairly recent light rainfall (a couple of inches in April-May), the countryside was tinted a pale green.

After Winnemucca there were no more climbs and descents, which in good measure accounted for the higher average mph I made on the way to Lovelock. Good weather, especially an easterly wind as I rode to the southwest, also was a factor.

Day 10 (59). Saturday, May 24. Worried about the possibility of strong southwest winds, I wanted to leave Lovelock as early as I could. But the Ramada's restaurant didn't open until 5:30, there were a lot of customers, and service was slow. Because of that, I didn't get on the road until 6:45. After a good start, 25 miles in two hours, I thought

I could make Fernley, about 60 miles from Lovelock, by noon. There were some scattered clouds in the sky, the remnants of last night's thundershowers in the Sierras and eastward into parts of Nevada. By 9 the clouds were gone, and it began to get warm.

At mile 22 a ridge had to be crossed and its steepness warranted the granny gear for a mile or so. At mile 30 another climb, not steep but long, almost five miles, and then another soon afterward that lasted for 2 ½ miles.

I was passing through an especially dry area of parched, gray soil and sparse vegetation. At mile 38 I noticed that the rear tire was partially flat. Unable to find an obvious source of a puncture, I pumped the tire up as much as I could. By now I was riding into a light headwind, and the temperature had risen well into the 80s. At mile 45 the tire had lost most of its air. Pumped it up again and continued riding. Not only did the wind begin to increase, the slow leak persisted and required pumping the tire at 50, 53, 55, and 59 miles, shortly before I reached East Fernley. The last ten miles of today's ride seemed to take forever.

In Fernley the first motel I tried was fully booked because of the Memorial Day weekend. But a Best Western down the road had an opening. Since the room wasn't ready, I went to a tire repair/sales place, where a young guy patched the tube and I removed another small piece of wire that had pierced both the tire and the tube. I had answered his questions about where I was going and, evidently impressed, after talking to the shop manager he told me there would be no charge. I went to a McDonald's for lunch, returned to the motel and, after a shower, was feeling great. Thinking that accommodations might be hard to get in Carson City this Memorial Day weekend, for the first time on this trip I called ahead to reserve a motel room.

63 miles = 3,305 total. This trip = 614

The United States is often the target of anger throughout much of the world, and when I was representing the United States abroad I saw many manifestations of this. But it is well to remember that now, as then, the anti-Americanism is directed at the U.S. government or, specifically, at certain U.S. foreign policies and actions. Apart from extremist groups, in general people usually harbor no anger toward Americans as such; in fact, in my years abroad time and again I experienced that there is a widespread residual liking of Americans. In part this is because, as my bicycle trip attested, by and large Americans are friendly and generous people.

The kindness that the young man and his boss in the tire shop in Fernley extended to me was just the latest of the many warm encounters I had with people along the way. Just about everywhere I stopped to buy something or to eat, people wanted know where I was going, where I had come from, and how long I'd been on the road, or asked other questions about the ride. Hardly ever was anyone unpleasant, and I never heard disparaging remarks. To be sure, sometimes people could not fathom why an old guy like me was doing what I was doing. That, of course, was understandable.

From the journal:

Day 11 (60). Sunday, May 25. My old nemesis, the wind, came back to bite me, hard, today. Slept in until 5:45. Opted for the motel's breakfast offering and had two bowls of cold cereal instead of making the long walk to the restaurant across the highway. The walk and getting breakfast there would have taken an hour or so, and I was worried that the later I got on the road the likelier I would run into a strong headwind. By 6:45 I had ridden two miles to the turnoff to US 95A, which would take me south 14 more miles to US 50 at Silver Springs. The sky was overcast with high clouds that kept the maximum temperature today below 80°. Once I reached Silver Springs and turned west on 50, I was met with a headwind that increased in velocity (up to 30 mph) as the day wore on. The next six miles were uphill.

At 25 miles from Fernley I saw a restaurant, only to find that it was deserted and boarded up, and so I plodded on, struggling with the west wind. The countryside was dry and, to my eye, devoid of interest. Because of the force of the wind, I had to stay in low gear. At times I was able to make just five or six mph on level ground and only four or even three mph on the grades. There were several of these, the longest of which was seven miles. Before I got to it, I came to a restaurant at mile 38 and had a big breakfast. Because of the wind, the seven-mile climb that began just after the small town of Dayton, 40 miles from my starting point this morning, was difficult. A sign along the way showed that the gain in elevation from Silver Springs had been over 1,000 feet. The wind and climbing hadn't worn me out, but I was tired and relieved to reach the outskirts of Carson City at about 2. The distance to the Best Western hotel/casino was another five miles and took 40 minutes.

If tomorrow morning the wind is still blowing as strongly from the west as it was this afternoon, I wonder whether I can make it over the mountains.

54 miles = 3,359 Total. This trip = 668

CHAPTER 11

Up and Over the Sierra Nevada and Down into California

Climb the mountains and get their good tidings.

John Muir

It's a mountain area with hills where you go like straight up, ... I mean, it's so steep in places you almost have to stop pedaling. I like that kind of stuff. Your chest just starts to burn from your heart beating so fast.

Reggie Brown

California, here I come, right back where I started from.

Buddy DeSylva and Joseph Meyer

I had heard that climbing over the Sierra Nevada would be more difficult than crossing the Rockies. And that, I found, was true. The ascent would be in two stages: the first up the Carson

Range—the spur of the Sierra Nevada between Carson City and Lake Tahoe—to Spooner Summit; the second from the lake up to Echo Summit. From Carson City's 4,730-foot elevation, I would climb 2,426 feet to Spooner's 7,156-foot elevation at the eastern rim of the bowl in which Tahoe sits, drop down 931 feet to the lake, ride to its other side and then go up 1,152 feet from there to Echo Summit at the bowl's western rim. The difficulty of the crossing lies not in the altitude, which was about 4,000 lower than Monarch Pass in the Rockies, but in the steepness of the two climbs.

Like the Appalachians and the Rockies, the Sierra Nevada arose as a result of tectonic uplifting many millions of years ago. It is the youngest of the three mountain ranges and is continuing to grow, especially on its eastern side. During California's rainy season, moisture-laden clouds roll in from the Pacific, and by the time they have risen over the crest of the Sierra Nevada they have been emptied of their rain and snow. As a result, the two sides of the mountains have substantially different landscapes—the west, for example, is more heavily forested than the much drier east.

From California's flat Central Valley and up through the Sierra's western foothills, the slopes rise gradually, in contrast to the steep escarpment of the eastern side, which plunges some 10,000 feet at its highest elevations to the floor of the Great Basin. John McPhee likens a cross section of the Sierra Nevada to a raised trapdoor or an airfoil or a woodshed with a long sloping back and a sheer front.[12] It is this abrupt steep rise in elevation from east to west that accounts for the toughness of the east-west bike ride up and over the Sierra Nevada.

---

12 John McPhee, *Assembling California* (New York: Farrar, Strauss, Giroux, 1981), 17, 18.

From a post-dinner addition to the May 25 journal:

A man in the casino bar tonight where I had a beer and lost a whole dollar on a 25-cent video poker game told me the wind on the road up to Lake Tahoe won't be like it is here in town. Hope he is right.

Day 12 (61). Monday, May 26. He was. No wind blowing when I left the hotel at 6:50. Rode south to the Tahoe turnoff and began to climb. Stopped to take a picture of the road, discovered I'd left my camera behind, rode back to the hotel, found the camera in a wastebasket, and started over again at 7:30. Conditions were good—only a light breeze later in the day and, for a few hours, an overcast that kept the maximum temperature below 80°.

The 9.4-mile climb to Spooner Summit (elev. 7,156 feet) *took a little over two hours. Occasionally I got up to 5 mph, but I chugged along at 4 mph most of the time, breathing hard all the way. It seemed to me that this was more physically demanding than the climb to Monarch Pass in the Rockies, even though Spooner is 4,000 feet lower in elevation. Near the beginning of the climb, before passing me, a guy on a racing bike who was out for a morning ride said Echo Summit would be a harder climb. After reaching Spooner, because a cool wind was blowing I put on my windbreaker, then coasted down a few miles to Lake Tahoe.*

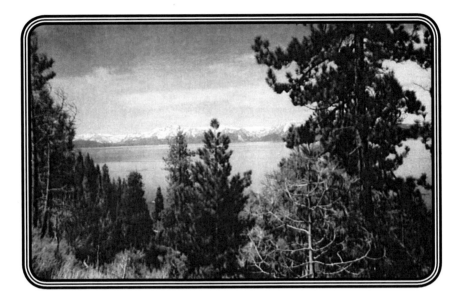

US 50 in the vicinity of the lake was packed with cars this Memorial Day. After stopping at noon for a sandwich at Zephyr Cove, I rode four miles or so to just beyond Stateline into South Lake Tahoe, California, where I took the Pioneer Trail and other back roads, keeping off US 50 for several miles until it headed up to Echo Summit. Began climbing around one o'clock. By now it was warm, and the 3.9 steep miles to the summit, about which I'd been warned this morning, were indeed tough.

The climb to Spooner Summit had taken some of the sap out of my legs, and to get to Echo Summit I really had to labor to keep going at just 4 mph. Anaerobic all the way, but I made it and was delighted to have crossed the Sierras.

The 25-mile downhill ride, steep at first then less so after a few miles, was great sport. A few miles before the descent ended, I stopped to talk to the driver of a large tow truck who was preparing to haul an RV that had conked out. He told me the first place I could find a motel would be Pollock Pines, about 15 miles farther west, and added that there would be an uphill of four or five miles. Unfortunately for me, this turned out to be a steep 5.3-mile grade that, because I was beginning to tire, was almost as much work for me as the two morning climbs had been. So I was more than pleased when I reached Pollack Pines.

After buying some bananas and Gatorade for tomorrow's ride, I was about to enter a steakhouse for supper, when a man standing in front of it said I'd do much better, at considerably less expense, if I went instead to hamburger joint a block away. Good advice, for the burger and (real) milkshake I had were great. Rode another two miles to the first motel I came to and, at 5 pm, called it a day.

I should note that from Silver Springs to Carson City, US 50 was not a bad road at all from a bicyclist's point of view: just two lanes but adequate shoulder width. That continued this morning until I got to Tahoe. There the shoulder narrowed to nothing at times, and it was a relief to get onto the Pioneer Trail. Going up to Echo Summit was okay, since generally I had two or three feet of shoulder. But after that, all the way to Pollack Pines there was either no shoulder or just a few inches of one, which created a few nerve wrenching moments as cars whizzed by. Worst was when RVs or cars pulling trailers passed, taking just about every inch of the lane and coming uncomfortably close.

83 miles = 3,442 total. This trip = 751

When I wrote in my journal that I labored during the four-mile climb to Echo Summit and that it was "anaerobic all the way," I was understating how hard it was for me. This was not a steady, endurance-type of activity like a long-distance run, but more of an all-out effort like a long sprint, say 400 meters. My heart rate was at its maximum and I was breathing hard all the way. I was intent on not stopping until I got to the top, in part simply because I wanted to meet the challenge and in part because the road was packed with cars and—ego again—I didn't want to fail in front of so many people. Anyway, I kept at it and I remember thinking that if ever my heart is going to give out because of extreme exertion, now is the time. The extra-hard work made reaching the summit all the sweeter.

It goes without saying that someone in his or her seventies, as I was, does not have the heart of a young person. But with regular exercise and reasonable eating habits, that fact needn't be too limiting.

During vigorous exercise, the muscles that are doing the work need more fuel in the form of oxygen via the circulatory system. Sad but true in old people, fit or unfit, less blood, and therefore less oxygen, reaches the muscles, adversely affecting performance. Interestingly, the diminished physical performance of people who are in good shape occurs as they age not because the maximum amount of blood pumped out with each heartbeat is lower, because in fact that volume is generally unchanged between ages 20 and 80.

In decades past, it was assumed that the heart weakened with age as its walls thinned. We now know, however, that the walls actually thicken with age. Scientists believe the increased thickness enables the heart walls to pump more strongly to cope with the greater stresses of aging, such as pumping blood through stiffer blood vessels. The normally stretchy tissue of major arteries is replaced by stiff, fibrous tissue, and the heart has to work harder to push blood through the less resilient vessels.

All of which leads to this question: If the volume of blood being pumped out per beat is not diminished with age, why do muscles of an older athlete or exerciser receive less oxygen during intense physical activity? The answer is that with age the maximal heart rate—the highest number of times the heart can contract per minute—decreases. The upshot of this is that during intense physical activity less oxygen gets to the working muscles of an older person than to those of a younger person. In addition, there's the age-related decrease in muscle mass. So it was that, for example, while riding up to Echo Summit I was stretched to the limit, an equally fit younger rider would have had an easier time of it. Nevertheless, by being in reasonably good physical condition, I was able to accomplish the climb.

The lesson, yet again, is that despite the normal declines in physical ability that come with aging, regular exercise pays big dividends.

From the journal:

Day 13 (62). Tuesday, May 27. Woke up at 5:30, but didn't get up for a while. I thought I had lots of time this morning because I was only riding to Sacramento, some 50 miles away. Also, I wanted to stop at a bicycle shop in Placerville, not far from Pollock Pines, and I figured the bike shop wouldn't be open until after 9. Breakfast in the motel was a bowl of cereal, cheese Danish, and coffee.

It was clear and almost warm, maybe 55°, when I left the motel at 8:25. Coasted a mile to US 50, now a freeway, then coasted another 5 ½ miles before the road leveled off. Arrived in Placerville, 11 miles from the motel, at 8:55 (average speed 22 mph—not too shabby for an old man on a loaded bicycle).

The bike shop was closed until 9:30, which gave me time for a full breakfast at a nearby café. At the bike shop some work needed to be done on the gear-shifting mechanism, and I bought another spare tube. Because US 50 is closed to bicycles from Placerville on, and perhaps even where I rode on it this morning, I got directions for an alternative route. Was also told how to get to the American River Parkway once I reached Folsom.

Back on the road by 10:30, with good reason to think that today's ride would be easy. There would be more downhill stretches on the way to Folsom and from there would be only a dozen or so miles of a level riding along the river to Sacramento. But this was not to be.

After passing through the picturesque gold rush town of Placerville, I found the entrance back to the freeway—on which it was legal to ride a bike for another half-mile—and proceeded to the exit for Green Valley Road, which would take me to Folsom. But right after taking the exit, I began encountering problems. Coming to the steepest rise I'd ever encountered on a bicycle, I struggled upward for several minutes until I reached the top. After that this country road rose and fell as it wound through the pretty country-side. Pines gave way to oaks, and the roadside was often lined with lupines and poppies. Definitely California countryside.

The road had no shoulder, and even though traffic was light, the passing cars and trucks occasionally came closer than I liked. I couldn't understand why it was so much hillier than I expected. At 12:15, 27 miles from Placerville, I learned that I had taken a wrong turn not far out of the town and was wandering around in a north-west direction instead of southwest toward Folsom. The error had cost me ten miles of extra work. I was given directions on how to get back to Green Valley Road, and soon was back on the right track,

Not long afterward, I stopped at a convenience store to buy some water. About four miles farther along, I opened my handlebar bag to get a banana and was aghast to find that my wallet was not in it. Only then did I remember that I had laid it on top of the rack over the rear wheel when I came out of the convenience store while I opened the handlebar bag before riding off. But, wonder of won-ders, luck was with me again, for there it was, right were I had put it.

Reached a T-junction at Folsom at 1:30 and, as instructed in a note on the map I'd been given at the bicycle shop in Placerville, turned left to ride the short distance to the entrance to American River Parkway bicycle trail. However, after 20 minutes and no sign of the river, I began to doubt I was on the right track. Even though I was passing through a densely populated area of tract housing, over half an hour went by before I managed to find a human be-ing outdoors who wasn't traveling in a car, a gardening service guy who told me that my directions were 180 degrees incorrect; I should *have turned right at the T-junction. So back I went and a few miles later, past the Folsom prison, I crossed Rainbow Bridge, which took me to the trail.*

It was now 2:40 and a hot 93°. A sign by the trail showed that I'd underestimated the distance to Sacramento from here, which instead of a dozen miles was 28. I was running out of water, but a few miles down the trail, I came upon the first of several water fountains. I drank my fill, poured water over my head, and rode on, enjoying the shade of the trees along the trail and the views of the river.

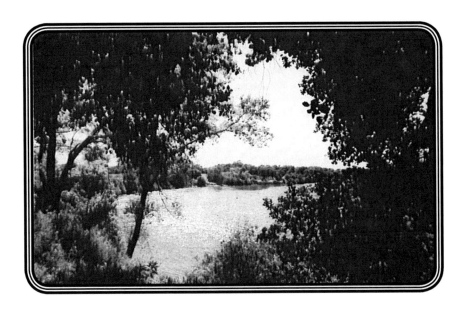

At 5:30 I came to the end of the American River Parkway. Called my cousin Nancy, who within minutes drove up and took me and the bike to her house. That night she, her husband John, two of their three children, John's mother, and I went to an excellent restaurant for dinner. I'm glad my route took me to Sacramento and enabled me to spend a wonderful evening with them. A bit after 10, dead tired,

I turned in. Before I got to Sacramento, the day had been frustrating, yet ultimately satisfying because I overcame unexpected misfortunes and reached my destination.

74 miles = 3,526 total. This trip = 825

Day 14 (63). Wednesday, May 28. At 8:15, after breakfast with the Drabble-Sims family, I rode downtown to West Capital Street, which took me to the bridge across the Sacramento River.

I made the crossing by riding on a bicycle/pedestrian path—at the outset right next to I-80 and terribly noisy—which continued to run adjacent to the highway over a causeway heading toward Davis. Riding on I-80 across Utah and Nevada, I had not been bothered by traffic noise, but here in California the volume of traffic was much, much heavier and commensurately the noise was much louder. After a few miles, however, the bike path deviated from I-80 and followed a frontage road into Davis, an attractive college town. Checked my tire pressure at a bike shop and ascertained that the detailed directions I had for getting to the Golden Gate were correct. Bought water and Gatorade and headed for Winters on a bike path that ended several miles later. Rode through the sort of rich agricultural country you would expect to find in California's Central Valley—groves of walnut, almond, and apricot trees and vast fields of tomatoes and other more recently sown crops.

Arrived in Winters at noon. Although a thermometer on a store-front registered 100°, the temperature actually was a mere 93°. The *heat provided evidence, if I needed any, that my decision to remain here for the afternoon and tonight was wise, especially since I learned after getting here that I would be facing an uphill ride to Lake Berryessa, about a dozen miles from Winters, and then another 25 miles or so of riding to reach Napa. In this heat, it made no sense at all to keep going. No motels or hotels in Winters, but the town's one bed and breakfast, which had just opened, had a room. A little pricey, at $89, but the room is commodious and pleasant. After showering, I had lunch at a restaurant around the corner, did my laundry at a Laundromat and bought water, Gatorade, and bananas at a grocery store.*

34 miles = 3,550 total. This trip = 859

A postscript: For dinner I went to the Buckhorn Steak and Roadhouse, two blocks away from my B&B. The restaurant was packed, and I soon discovered why—the food was superb. Talked to the owner, who told me that people, attracted by the restaurant's reputation, come from all around the area and from farther away. During our conversation I told him how as a child I had passed through Winters with my parents and brothers on our way from Pismo Beach to visit my grandparents in Chico. Also told him about my current trip. He asked me to send him a letter about the rest of the ride. Later, after I'd given my credit card to my waitress, she returned to tell me the meal was on the house.

As I got to lower elevations in the foothills, the countryside took on the characteristics that are so familiar to Californians. Rolling hills, which for a good half of the year display the state's distinctive yellow-brown dryness, were still green from the tail end of the rainy season and speckled with trees, mainly live oaks, which are native to the state and are among the most common of California's trees. Poppies and lupines were abundant and reminded me of childhood explorations in the hills and fields around Pismo Beach.

Having reached Winters, I was now close to the western limit of the great Central Valley, which dominates the central part of the state, typically 40 to 60 miles wide and running some 450 miles north to south from the Cascade Range to the Tehachapi Mountains. Once an inland sea, the valley is about as flat as any part of the earth can be, certainly flatter than Kansas. The most productive agricultural area of California, it is one of the most productive in the world as well. Riding past orchards and fields, I had an overwhelming sense of how fertile this land is. Summers in the valley can be brutally hot, and the 93° temperature on this day in late May was nothing unusual.

The next day's ride would take me into part of the Coastal Range. No formidable climbs in store, but headwinds would ensure that this segment of the trip would not be easy.

From the journal:

Day 15 (64). Thursday, May 29. It must have been about 60° when, at 7:15, I rode west out of Winters on California Rte 128, headed for Lake Berryessa. After nine miles, I made the one-mile steep climb to the lake. For another four miles the road continued upward, but less steeply. A westerly wind slowed me but had a cooling effect and kept the flies at bay. At mile 17 there was another upslope, this one for two miles. At 20 miles, I took a fork in the road that led through hills to Napa. Passed by oak trees festooned in clumps of moss hanging from branches. The road rose and fell, but mostly rose. At 10:30 the wind increased sharply; it would continue to blow from the west-southwest all day long. At 26 miles I turned onto Rte 121. By now the wind was so strong that I could only average 4 mph. Finally, though, the road began to descend and I coasted 3.5 miles to the outskirts of Napa. Pedaled through town, stopping for a hamburger at a Jack-in-the-Box.

Sought directions to Petaluma and was advised to take CA Rte 29, which I did, only to discover that it is closed to bicycles. Once off 29, I got new directions, which put me on a bike path that paralleled the highway for a few miles until Rte 121 came into play again where it branches off 29 and heads west. The temperature had stopped rising by mid-morning and then began dropping. Today's maximum temperature was about 60°, a huge difference from yesterday's 93° in Winters.

There were more hills to climb on California routes 121, 12 and 116. All three roads kept me on a westerly course, generally directly into the wind. And on all three the shoulders ranged from very narrow to non-existent. At mile 58, just before turning north to go into Petaluma, I talked to two men at a saloon-cum-car repair shop. One of them, a cyclist, asked me where I was coming from. When I told him Napa, he said that the roads I came on were extremely dangerous riding and that he never rode on them anymore. Seems I find out about dangerous roads only after I've finished riding on them.

Now that I had turned away from the headwind, I made the remaining several miles into the center of Petaluma in good time. Arrived at 5. It had taken me almost ten hours to ride 64 miles. Not an easy day.

64 miles = 3,614 total. This trip = 923

CHAPTER 12

The Last Day

I fell in love with the most cordial and sociable city in the Union.

Mark Twain

East is East, and West is San Francisco

O. Henry

The Bay Area is so beautiful, I hesitate to preach about heaven while I'm here.

Billy Graham

From the journal:

Day 16 (65). Friday, May 30. The morning started with a typical coastal California high fog, whose chill dictated that I wear my rain pants. At 7:45 I left Petaluma on D Street, which became Point

*Reyes/Petaluma Road. The first hill I came to warmed me up to such
an extent that I shed the pants and my windbreaker as well. This hill,
a mile in length, was followed soon afterward by another, a mile and
a half long and quite steep. I was working harder than I expected
on this last day of the trip, but because there was no headwind, I
couldn't complain. Riding in a southwesterly direction, I was looking
for Nicasio Valley Road, which would take me to Sir Francis Drake
Boulevard to Fairfax and other towns on the way to San Francisco,
an alternate route to US 101, which is closed to bicycles. At about
mile ten, coming down a hill I saw Nicasio on a road sign, or so I
thought, and turned left on a wonderful road, flat or slightly downhill, that passed through gorgeous green countryside, and I figured I'd
reach the Golden Gate in no time at all. But when, nine miles later,
I entered the town of Novato, well to the east of where I was supposed
to be, I asked at a gas station and learned I'd taken Novato Road, not
Nicasio Valley Road. Bonehead!*

*Facing the prospect of a nine-mile mainly uphill backtrack, I must
have looked beseechingly at a guy in a pickup who was headed that
way. He made a U-turn and pulled up to where I was standing. He
said he had thought I was a bicycling friend of his, but readily agreed
to take me to Point Reyes/Petaluma Road. Driving at about 75 mph
on the country road, he scared the hell out of me. Once there, at
10:50, I rode about three miles farther west to Nicasio Valley Road.
(Because we were backtracking, I don't consider these three miles or,
of course, the ride in the pickup as having anything to do with the
mileage of today's ride.)*

*About ten miles later I came to Sir Francis Drake Boulevard.
Soon the traffic got to be heavy, and I was thankful to find a bicycle
path. Stopped for a hot dog and milk shake at 12:30 in the town of*

Fairfax. From there I rode to San Anselmo and Kentfield, where the bike path ended and I found myself back on Sir Francis Drake Blvd, where the heavy traffic made riding this street too dicey for my taste. Two policemen whose advice I sought told me to go back a half mile and turn west for a couple of blocks to Magnolia Street, which parallels SFD Blvd but carries far fewer cars. That indeed was so, but they neglected to tell me that the street climbs steeply up the high hillside that runs along the western edge of the valley through which the roads running south toward San Francisco pass. I guess it was meant to be that there would one last tough hill near the end of my ride. But with it came the reward of a steep downhill for a couple of miles. When it ended at an intersection, I turned left for two blocks, entered the San Francisco Bay Trail, and followed it as it skirted the bay going into Sausalito.

I had been in touch with my daughter Susan and son Brian by cell phone, and they, my granddaughter Jadyn (Susan's daughter), Susan's partner, John Lyddon, and his son Brendon met me at a small park in town with a warm welcome, congratulations, and hugs and kisses.

Only a couple of miles to go. We left the park in Sausalito at about 3, riding on Bridgeway, the street that leads to the bridge. As they drove in their car, before leaving me to take 101 across the bridge, they filmed and photographed me as I rode along. One final climb, a few blocks long. Cresting the hill, I saw, at long last, the beautiful Golden Gate.

Bridgeway took me to a bicycle lane that in turn led onto the bicycle/pedestrian lane on the bay (east) side of the bridge. After stopping to take a picture, elated to have finished what I started out to do, I rode onto and across the bridge, where Susan, John, Brian, and the kids met me again.

And there my journey ended.

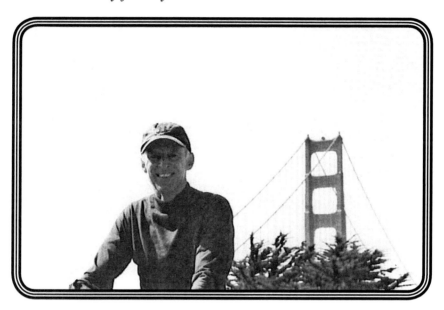

54 miles = 3,668 total. This trip = 977

It took me 65 days to complete the journey. Days off because of weather, muscle cramps, or a needed brake repair and boil lancing accounted for six of those days, leaving a total of 59 days on the road for an average of 62 miles a day. That would have been higher if I hadn't ended several rides early to be sure of getting a motel close by a restaurant. In any event, I figured that the 62-mile average on a loaded touring bike wasn't too bad for an old guy.

It's not often that the visible handiworks of human beings are improvements over their natural surroundings. The Golden Gate Bridge is an exception to the rule, as any pictures of the Golden Gate Strait before and after construction of the bridge graphically attest. The span linking Fort Point on the San Francisco side to the Marin headland was built in Art Deco style and painted orange vermillion because the color was considered a warm hue consistent with the warm colors of the land and distinct from the cool colors of sea and sky. It was an excellent choice. The bridge is a magnificent, singular creation that adds greatly to the beauty of San Francisco Bay. When I was in the navy, one of the ships I served on passed beneath the bridge many times. Each passage was a glorious experience.

I could have cut a day off my trip if I had ridden to Vallejo in the East Bay and taken a ferry to San Francisco. And I would have avoided the difficulties I had during the ride from Winters to Petaluma. But from the beginning my goal was to ride to and across the Golden Gate Bridge. Accomplishing that was to me a fitting climax to the cross-country adventure.

Since the accident at Price and also a bout with pneumonia in 2010 that put me in an intensive care unit for five days, I have had a greater appreciation of what I feel are the good things in life, such as family, friendships, a beautiful sky, the pristine white coating of the land just after a snowfall, a brilliant sunrise or sunset, music, works of art, books, films, and other natural and man-made wonders. This kind of high-mindedness is not with me all the time, not in a world that is far from free of heart-wrenching disasters and great disappointments, but it helps come to terms with them. And although I have moments of pettiness or anger, they quickly pass as my equanimity reasserts itself.

Completing the ride was a reminder, which I hope has influenced loved ones and friends, that it is good once in a while to push the envelope if only a little bit, to be willing to break away from the ordinary and to try to do something that in one way or another puts you to a test. At times I recall an incident of my across-America journey and I say to myself, "That was hard, and, doggone it, I did it." A moment of honest pride never hurt anyone.

Epilogue

A year later, I rode 2,011 miles from Miami to New Hampshire. This solo ride up the East Coast was less work than my east-west cross-country trek and not as rewarding. Which is not to say it was either easy or uneventful. From Miami Beach well into New Jersey the terrain was essentially flat, and for most of the ride I didn't suffer from headwinds, as I did during a good portion of the NH-San Francisco trip. But some hot and humid weather, at times bicycle-unfriendly roads, and occasional hazardous traffic conditions added up to some difficulty. These were more than balanced by the enjoyment of seeing a good chunk of the country that I had not seen before—Florida's east coast, eastern parts of Georgia and South Carolina, North Carolina's Outer Banks, some rural areas of New Jersey, and many miles along or near the Delaware River. Although the scenery lacked the grandeur of the American West, every day something interesting took place and every day had moments of scenic beauty. This trip was not purely self-indulgent (if you can call long-distance bike riding self-indulgence), because I was riding for a cause—to help promote campaign finance reform.

In early 2012 I began thinking seriously about making another cross-country ride, this time from west to east. I even planned a route that would take me from Los Angeles to Phoenix, through southern Arizona and New Mexico to El Paso; east-southeast to Austin and on to southern Louisiana, southernmost Mississippi and Alabama; over to Pensacola, Gainesville, and Jacksonville, Florida; then north to Georgia, eastern South Carolina, the Outer Banks of North Carolina, and on to Richmond, Virginia, and Washington, DC.

What led me to want to try to make the ride again? First, I was committed to the effort to bring about campaign finance reform. Perhaps, I thought, an over-80-year-old former US ambassador plodding across the US on a bicycle might draw some attention, which I could milk for publicity for the need to reform the financing of federal elections. Second, I wanted to see how it would be to ride from west to east. And third was the lure of another adventure. Time, of course, had softened remembrances of the stresses and strains, and pains, of the 2002 trip.

For me, February was much too cold for bicycling in New Hampshire, so I had my touring bike boxed up and, accompanied by Julie, took it to San Francisco. We stayed with my daughter Susan and John at their home in the hills high above Half Moon Bay, where I took the bike each day for rides on California Rte 1. This sector of the highway, which parallels the Pacific, rising and falling with its cliffs, mixes moderate and steep climbs with level stretches, a perfect combination for training rides. Increasing my mileage each day, after about ten days I had managed a ride of 60 miles, but it wore me to a frazzle. A few more rides led me to conclude that it was most unlikely I could manage to ride from Los Angeles to Washington, DC on a loaded touring bike.

Some more practice rides after I had returned to New Hampshire only added more weight to that judgment. Physical realities could not be denied. The nine years since I had ridden from Miami home to Brentwood, New Hampshire, had taken their inevitable toll. For instance, in that time my body's muscle mass must have decreased significantly, robbing my leg muscles of the strength I would need to ride long distances day after day. No doubt the efficiency of my circulatory system had also diminished.

Of course I'm disappointed not to be able to make the ride. But I have to keep the disappointment in perspective. Considering the full range of bad things that can happen in life, this has been no more than a very minor setback. Furthermore, perhaps it's for the best: If I had been able to undertake the journey, perhaps I would have been undone by the flu or another illness, or some other major problem could have arisen and scuttled the attempt.

In any event, my health is good and my wonderful wife, children, and grandchildren continue to put up with my idiosyncrasies.

Index

flat tires (punctures), 104, 164, 191,
    193
flying, 18, 21-23
    See also ultra-light aircraft
Friedan, Betty, 12-13

Gatorade, 114-115, 138
glaciation (ice age), 6, 118
Golden Gate. *See* San Francisco
    Golden Gate Bridge
Grain silos and elevators, 122
Great Basin Desert, 150, 186
Great Plains, 117-118, 119
    rural population, decline of, 126
Great Salt Lake Desert, 170-172,
    186

headwinds, strong, *See* Winds
health problems, 10
    obesity and, 9-10
    tobacco usage and, 10, 13
heart. *See* aging
heat
    body's reaction to, 90
    and the elderly, 90-91, 135
heat exhaustion, 90, 92, 135
heat index, 90-91
hitchhiking, 92, 93-94, 112
homing instinct, 19-20
hot weather. *See* weather
Humboldt River, 179-180

Ice Age. *See* glaciation
immune system. *See* aging
interstate highways
    advantages of riding on, 152
    See also US interstate routes by
        number

joints. *See* aging

Kansas, 107
    countryside, 118, 122
    Flint Hills, 118
    Great Bend, 119, 127
    Kansas Rte 96, 121, 125
    McPherson, 114 127
    Ness City, 121, 127
    Scott City,124, 127
    settlement of, 126-127
    terrain of, 109, 117, 128
    Tribune, 126, 127
Keller, Helen, 15
knee pain ("runner's knee"), 177

Lake Erie, 61, 63
Lake Tahoe, 199-200
leg cramps, 87-88, 119, 120
    See also muscle fatigue
lightning, danger to cyclists of, 124,
    125
lungs. *See* aging

maps, 97
McCurdy, Bruce, 24-25, 111
McPhee, John, 180, 198
Mencken, H.L., 79
Merritt, Bill and Andy, 121
"Metaphor: The Tree of Life",
    See Utah
Miami to New Hampshire ride, 219
Midwest, The, 78-79
Mississippi River, 95-97
Missouri
    Chillicothe, 102
    Hannibal, 96, 97
    Macon, 99
    St. Joseph, 105
    Shelbina, 98
motels, quality of, 110, 120
muscle, *See also* aging
    fatigue, 51, 75, 83-84, 85-86

CPSIA information can be obtained at www.ICGtesting.com
Printed in the USA
BVOW02s1122050716

453904BV00010BA/218/P